OUTSMART DIABETES

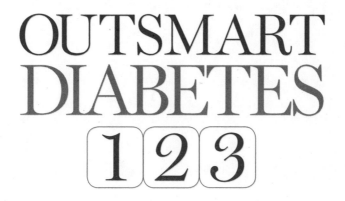

123

OUTSMART DIABETES

1 2 3

- ■ Beat the odds of developing complications

- ■ Change the lifestyle factors that compromise blood sugar control

- ■ Diabetes-proof your body for a long, vital life

BY THE EDITORS OF **Prevention**.

RODALE

Prevention is a registered trademark of Rodale Inc.

Printed in the United States of America

Book design by Carol Angstadt
Cover photographs (left to right): © Russell Sadur/Getty Images; © Alison Miksch/Brand X Pictures; © Stockbyte/Getty Images

Contributing writers: Nicole Nader Gabor, Doug Hill, Eric Metcalf, Wyatt Myers, Kathy Summers, Marie Suszynski, Julia VanTine-Reichardt

ISBN-13: 978-1-60529-865-8

RODALE
LIVE YOUR WHOLE LIFE™

CONTENTS

HOW TO USE THIS BOOK.. viii

Introduction: Understanding Diabetes

You're Not Alone 3

The Many Faces of Diabetes 14

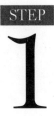

STEP 1

Outsmart Diabetes Complications

FROM HEAD TO TOE

Vision Problems (Retinopathy) 27

Gum Disease... 36

Heart Disease... 44

High Blood Pressure 52

Kidney Disease... 61

Liver Disease 69

Urinary Incontinence.. 76

Erectile Dysfunction 83

Peripheral Arterial Disease.............................. 94

Foot Complications.. 105

WHOLE-BODY COMPLICATIONS

Hypoglycemia... 116

Diabetic Neuropathy 125

Polycystic Ovary Syndrome.............................. 140

Stroke.. 147

STEP 2

Navigate the Diabetes Danger Zones

Abdominal Fat 157
Dining Out 164
Environmental Exposure 170
Lack of Exercise 176
Lack of Sleep 184
Overweight 192
Skipping Meals 201
Smoking 206
Stress 213
Sweet Tooth 219
Traveling 226

STEP 3

Diabetes-Proof Your Life

1. Know Your Risk 235
2. Monitor Your Blood Sugar 241
3. Get Regular Screenings 249
4. Follow Prescriptions to the Letter 257
5. Trim Your Waistline 269
6. Get the Healthiest Mix of Carbs, Protein, Fat, and Fiber 278
7. Take Advantage of Diabetes-Friendly Foods 289
8. Use Supplements Sensibly 302
9. Make Exercise an Everyday Event 314
10. Adopt a Positive "Diatitude" 327

INDEX 336

How to Use This Book

DIABETES ought to come with its own instruction manual.

The diagnosis can be confusing enough; just what is diabetes anyway? More to the point, once you've got it, how do you keep it in check?

Answering these questions could easily, well, fill a book. This one is the culmination of hundreds of hours of interviewing experts and scouring the scientific literature, driven by a singular objective: to empower you and others who have diabetes not just to live *with* the disease, but to live *beyond* it—that is, to manage it so effectively that it has the least possible impact on your long-term health and quality of life.

It's true that diabetes isn't curable—at least not yet. But as we learned from doctors, nurses, nutritionists, exercise physiologists, certified diabetes educators (CDEs), and other professionals who specialize in diabetes care, the disease is treatable and controllable. In the case of type 2, by far the most common form of diabetes (and our primary focus here), this usually means lifestyle changes, possibly in combination with medication—though it's worth noting that maintaining a healthy lifestyle can delay and even eliminate the need for drug therapy.

Of course, maintaining a healthy lifestyle takes effort. Even the most vigilant among us will have moments when our self-care gets a little lax. The trouble is, high blood sugar can start doing damage—the kind that leads to diabetes complications—long before diabetes is even diagnosed.

That's the reality check. But the opposite is also true: You can lower your risk of complications by stabilizing your blood sugar at a healthy level. The pages that follow provide plenty of nuts-and-bolts advice about nutrition, exercise, weight loss, sleep, stress reduction, and the myriad other factors that influence your blood sugar, along with an ample dose of encouragement and reassurance to help you stay on track.

For ease of use, we've organized this book into four sections. The introduction, Understanding Diabetes, provides a comprehensive overview of diabetes—its prevalence, its most common forms, and its whole-body effects. Whether you're newly diagnosed or you're well into treatment, these chapters will give you a clear picture of the "state of the science" in diabetes management.

In Step 1, Outsmart Diabetes Complications, we take a closer look at how this one disease can contribute to other health problems—quite literally, from head to toe. Here you can assess your risk of the most common complications and learn strategies for slowing and possibly reversing any diabetes-related damage.

This leads us to Step 2, Navigate the Diabetes Danger Zones. You probably already know how your eating habits and your activity level can cause spikes and dips in your blood sugar readings. But did you know that stress, lack of sleep, and even your mood can influence both your blood sugar level and your ability to bring it into balance? Here we'll explore how these and other lifestyle factors can undermine diabetes management and what you can do to shore up your self-care efforts.

Step 3, Diabetes-Proof Your Life, presents the 10 fundamental principles that collectively can help ensure optimal diabetes control. Incorporate these guidelines into your lifestyle, and you can stave off the disease's more insidious effects and lay the foundation for a long, vital life.

This is what we mean when we talk about outsmarting diabetes: Armed with the most reliable information and the best tools, you can stay a step ahead of the disease. So let's get started!

UNDERSTANDING DIABETES

You're Not Alone

IT'S A RAINY SATURDAY MORNING IN NOVEMBER, and about 100 people are sitting in the auditorium of Mountainside Hospital in Montclair, New Jersey. They've come to learn about diabetes.

At the moment, the hospital's head of psychiatric services, Edward Latimer, MD, is onstage, discussing some of the emotional issues associated with diabetes. People who are recently diagnosed with the disease, he says, often go through the same stages of grief as someone who has experienced a deep personal loss: denial, anger, bargaining, depression, and, finally, acceptance.

Dr. Latimer opened his talk by explaining that he likes to engage his audiences in dialogue. True to his word, he interrupts his presentation to throw out a question to the crowd.

"What's depressing about diabetes?" he asks.

Only a moment passes before hands raise and voices ring out in the darkened auditorium.

"You have to stick yourself all the time," a woman near the back says.

"You have to turn down food when you eat at somebody's house and try to explain to them that it isn't because you don't like what they cooked," says the man seated next to her.

"The routine," says a woman near the front. "Monitor, monitor, monitor.

Watch this, watch that, don't eat this, don't eat that. It gets old after a while."

Another woman near the back shouts, "The reactions of other people when they find out you have it!"

An older woman with a cane, seated on the aisle, speaks quietly, and Dr. Latimer asks her to repeat her comment.

"I'm always worried about what's next," she says. "What's coming in the future?"

Each of these comments is greeted with knowing nods of agreement and understanding around the auditorium.

Then Dr. Latimer calls on a man near the back of the room who's been waving his hand. "What's wrong with diabetes?" the man asks. "Everything!"

The whole audience laughs and nods.

If you've been diagnosed with diabetes, you might be imagining yourself in that auditorium in New Jersey, empathizing with the comments of those around you and perhaps throwing out one or two of your own. It's true that the prospect of living with diabetes seems daunting at times. It's also true, as that spontaneous group therapy session illustrates, that many people share the same fears and frustrations about the disease.

What the audience learned from Dr. Latimer and the other doctors, nurses, and nutritionists who spoke that day is that there are ways to keep diabetes from disrupting their lives. They learned that there are strategies to effectively control the disease and limit its impact on their overall health and vitality. They learned, in other words, that there is hope.

We created this resource for you, offering insight and guidance from dozens of health professionals who specialize in diabetes management, because we, too, believe that you can outsmart diabetes. Yes, it's a serious disease, but with proper self-care measures, you can minimize its effects on your body as well as your lifestyle. We'll show you how.

But first, let's take a closer look at the numbers behind diabetes. As you'll soon see, it's touching people of all stripes—young and old, male and female, all ethnicities, all incomes. Its implications for us, both as individuals and as a nation, have made it one of our most urgent health priorities for the early 21st century.

Diabetes by the Numbers

In public health circles these days, it's rare to hear a mention of diabetes without the word *epidemic* following close behind. A sampling of the statistics gives us a sense of the scope and depth of the problem.

- Currently, more than 20 million American adults and children have diabetes. That's about 7 percent of the US population.

- Between 1990 and 2000, the prevalence of diabetes in the United States jumped by nearly 50 percent.

- By 2050, prevalence is expected to more than double, with more than 48 million Americans being diagnosed with the disease.

- An American woman has a 38 percent chance of developing diabetes in her lifetime; an American man, 33 percent.

- Certain ethnic groups are more prone to diabetes than others. The disease is about twice as prevalent among non-Hispanic blacks and Mexican Americans as among non-Hispanic whites. As many as 3.2 million non-Hispanic blacks and 2.5 million Hispanic/Latino Americans already have diabetes.

- A growing number of children and adolescents are being diagnosed with type 2 diabetes, which the medical community long believed affected only people who were middle-aged or older (hence its former name, adult-onset diabetes). According to several clinical trials, the number of children with type 2 diabetes has climbed from less than 5 percent in 1994 to between 30 and 50 percent today—a trend that's commonly attributed to the growing rate of obesity among our younger generation.

- As many as 54 million Americans are prediabetic, which means that their higher-than-normal blood sugar levels predict a strong likelihood of developing type 2 diabetes—unless they lose weight and step up their physical activity.

- As of 2002, an estimated $132 billion of our nation's total medical expenditures was in some way attributable to diabetes, including $92 billion for direct medical care.

- Approximately one-third of all Medicare expenses go toward treating diabetes and its complications.

- According to the International Diabetes Federation, some 246 million adults worldwide have diabetes. That figure is expected to rise to 380 million by 2025. The president of the federation, Martin Silink, MD, told the *New York Times* that diabetes is "one of the biggest health catastrophes the world has ever seen."

One reason that Dr. Silink and other public health officials are so alarmed by statistics like these is that their predictions about diabetes, which once seemed over the top, may have been far too conservative. Back in 2003, for example, the Centers for Disease Control and Prevention (CDC) projected that the number of Americans diagnosed with diabetes would reach 39 million by 2050. Just 3 years later, the CDC revised that figure upward, by more than 9 million. In 2006, the World Health Organization (WHO) predicted that worldwide prevalence of diabetes would increase by 60 percent between 1995 and 2030. Just a year later, a Canadian study found that the disease's prevalence in Ontario already had grown by 60 percent between 1995 and 2005. Though admittedly this statistic is for just one Canadian province, it suggests that diabetes will surpass the WHO numbers much sooner than expected.

These statistical trends no longer surprise Larry Deeb, MD, a past president of the American Diabetes Association. In 1980, he was running numbers on diabetes for the CDC. Back then, there were 6 million cases of diabetes in the

United States, but the prevalence already was on the rise. Dr. Deeb's team predicted 21 million cases by 2010, which then seemed an almost unattainable number. In fact, we're already closing in on it, with a couple of years to spare. "Every time we predict a number," Dr. Deeb sighs, "it ends up being an underestimation."

The Story behind the Statistics

The reasons for the diabetes explosion in the United States and around the world are not especially mysterious. Nor, for that matter, are all of them bad.

In this country, for example, type 2 diabetes is becoming more common in large part because more of us Americans are living longer than we once did. With the first baby boomers already past their 60th birthdays, our older population is just beginning its growth spurt. The larger this population becomes, the more type 2 diabetes we'll see, because type 2, which accounts for 90 to 95 percent of all diabetes cases, most often develops in older people (although, as mentioned earlier, it also strikes the young).

Another demographic trend that's contributing to the surge in diabetes is the growth of our Hispanic population. As of 2006, those of Hispanic origin—who are at higher risk for the disease—accounted for 15 percent of the total US population.

The increase in diabetes isn't all about demographic shifts, however. We're also seeing more diabetes diagnoses because the medical community understands the disease much better and is able to identify it much earlier than ever before. Organizations such as the American Diabetes Association have aided the effort by increasing public awareness of diabetes. As a result, says Ann Albright, PhD, RD, director of the CDC's Division of Diabetes Translation, the number of people who have diabetes but don't know it has dropped from about half of all cases to about a third. That's a good thing, because the sooner a person with diabetes gets a proper diagnosis, the sooner he or she can begin treatment and gain an upper hand on the disease.

The "Diabesity" Lifestyle

Of course, the above factors don't explain exactly why so many of us Americans are becoming diabetic. Though the cause of type 1 diabetes remains something of a mystery (which we'll discuss further in the next chapter), experts generally peg type 2 diabetes as a lifestyle disease brought on by too many pounds and too little physical activity.

Obesity is a major risk factor for type 2 diabetes. The two have such a strong connection, in fact, that experts sometimes refer to them by a single term: *diabesity*. Obesity—like diabetes—is reaching epidemic proportions in the United States and throughout the world. And more often than not, it's a consequence of our modern lifestyle.

Think about it: Many of us spend our days sitting at desks or standing on assembly lines rather than plowing and planting fields. We eat burgers and fries from the drive-thru instead of fresh fruits and vegetables from the garden. We drive our cars to run errands rather than walking to the bank or the post office. All of these lifestyle changes are invitations to obesity and type 2 diabetes.

You're likely well aware that being overweight and out of shape is unhealthy, but let's take a moment to explore just why these two lifestyle factors have been implicated as the primary culprits behind our nation's diabetes epidemic.

First, while physical inactivity definitely increases the likelihood of weight gain, it also is an independent risk factor for type 2 diabetes. In other words, just being sedentary increases your chances of becoming diabetic, whether or not you're overweight. Combine inactivity and obesity, and you have a real double whammy for your diabetes risk.

For proof, consider the findings of a recent study involving 68,907 female nurses. Researchers analyzing the study data concluded that women who are obese and inactive are 16 times more likely to develop type 2 diabetes than those who are neither obese nor inactive. Women who are obese but active, on the other hand, have 10 times the risk.

Second, physical inactivity and weight gain contribute to type 2 diabetes by promoting the accumulation of body fat. It's long been thought that body fat is more or less an inert mass of stuff—unattractive, perhaps, but not particularly harmful. Now we know otherwise. Body fat is actually an engine of metabolic activity, and much of that activity is fueling our diabetes risk.

THE HISTORY OF DIABETES: IT'S A LONG STORY

Though the number of people with diabetes is exploding, the disease itself is far from new. In fact, it's been a recognized medical problem for much of human history. In the centuries before microscopic science, it was usually identified by one of its more obvious outward symptoms: excessive, sugary urination.

An Egyptian medical text known as the *Ebers Papyrus,* thought to have been written in about 1550 BC, describes the symptom of "passing too much urine"—almost certainly a sign of diabetes. When archeologists recently identified a mummy as the remains of Queen Hatshepsut, one of Egypt's most powerful rulers, the evidence from her obese corpse suggested that she may have been laid low by diabetes, among other diseases. Interestingly, modern Egypt is one of many countries where diabetes has reached epidemic proportions.

Hindu writings thousands of years old describe how ants and flies were attracted to the sugary urine of those with diabetes, a phenomenon also noted by the Indian physician Sushruta in 400 BC. But the disease didn't get its common name until the 2nd century BC, when the physician Aretaeus of Cappadocia wrote of how the organs of people afflicted with the malady seemed to liquefy and pass out of their bodies in their urine—hence the name *diabetes,* which is Greek for "siphon" or "pass through."

The medical term *diabetes mellitus* entered the lexicon much later, in 1674. Once again, sugary urine played a role in the naming process. Thomas Willis, a personal physician to King Charles II of England, noted that the urine of those with diabetes tasted as if it were "imbued with honey and sugar." Just how Willis came to this conclusion we'd rather not know. But we do know this: *Mellitus* is Latin for "honey."

For example, fat releases inflammatory substances into the bloodstream that can interfere with the hormone insulin. We'll discuss insulin at length in the next chapter; for now, suffice it to say that how our bodies make and use the hormone is a critical factor in whether or not we develop diabetes.

According to Francine R. Kaufman, MD, a past president of the American Diabetes Association and author of *Diabesity: The Obesity-Diabetes Epidemic That Threatens America—And What We Must Do to Stop It*, the fat that accumulates around our waistlines—called visceral fat—is especially suspect. That's because it tends to spill fat molecules, along with other harmful chemicals, into the body's tissues. Once on the loose, these fat molecules also hamper the body's production of insulin and the cells' response to it. The net result is what researchers call a physiological cascade—a biochemical downward spiral that ultimately ends in type 2 diabetes, perhaps in tandem with cardiovascular disease.

Into the Future

If type 2 diabetes is a lifestyle disease—a disease of progress, as Dr. Deeb describes it—can we realistically do anything to stop its march toward epidemic status? After all, most of us aren't about to give up the conveniences that modern life has bestowed upon us, even if that lifestyle means a thicker waistline and an elevated diabetes risk. As Dr. Deeb observes, "Progress means that the world is becoming a better place to live for a lot of people. But the things that make the world a better place to live are the same things that tend to bring out diabetes."

That said, diabetes is not inevitable, nor is it invincible. Habits and behaviors of modern life make us more vulnerable to the disease, but knowledge and technology make us better prepared to fight it. On the frontline of the battle are the physicians and scientists who are collaborating on medical advances that one day will transform how we diagnose and treat diabetes—and possibly lead to a cure. Beside them are the public health officials and nonprofit health organizations, which together have mobilized significant resources for diabetes research. Though some critics may argue that not enough is being done, even they likely will agree that diabetes awareness is at an all-time high.

Already we're seeing the fruits of this focused, all-out effort. New medications to help treat diabetes are making their debuts, with additional ones waiting in the wings. With new instruments and techniques, surgical treatments are becoming safer and more effective. New methods of blood sugar monitoring and insulin delivery are redefining self-care so that it's more personal and more precise than ever before.

And all this is just the proverbial tip of the iceberg. Teams of scientists around the country are working feverishly to understand why certain people are at higher risk for diabetes than others, including the isolation of possible diabetes "genes." The goal is to find ways to help people who are predisposed to diabetes avoid getting it in the first place.

THE THRIFTY GENE HYPOTHESIS

Has evolution programmed us humans for diabetes? A growing number of scientists believe that the answer to this question is yes. The so-called thrifty gene hypothesis holds that our hunter-gatherer ancestors routinely experienced extended periods when they didn't have much to eat. Those who were fattest tended to survive these famines because they carried built-in reserves of nourishment in their bellies. Over time, evolution favored humans with thrifty metabolisms, meaning a genetic tendency to store fat rather than burn it.

According to the hypothesis, the thrifty gene has been passed down to us over thousands of years. But times have changed, and this genetic adaptation actually threatens our survival rather than improving our odds. In developed countries, at least, there's plenty of food—perhaps too much—and virtually no need to hunt or gather. So the thrifty gene that protected us in leaner times now predisposes us to obesity and, therefore, to diabetes.

This takes us back to the role of lifestyle. We tend to think of "lifestyle" as diet and exercise, but it encompasses so much more, including social and cultural issues. To illustrate this point, Dr. Deeb describes how the entire structure of modern society is contributing to our national propensity toward overweight and obesity. "Sure, losing weight is a personal responsibility, and we need to remind people of that," he says. "But just as important, we as a society need to do what we can to make weight loss possible. When we design communities with no sidewalks; when we allow school cafeterias to serve junk food; when we have inner-city neighborhoods without access to fresh produce . . . whose responsibility is that?" Government officials at all levels are exploring these sorts of questions, with an eye toward instituting new programs and policies to address them. According to Dr. Albright, it means retooling our health care system—which is best equipped to address acute medical problems such as heart attacks and broken bones—to support chronic conditions, including diabetes. These conditions require ongoing care and management, which in turn requires a broader base of public and private services.

As director of the CDC's Division of Diabetes Translation, Dr. Albright is responsible for taking the findings of clinical studies and "translating" them into programs that reach people where they live. The ingrained cultural habits that feed into diabetes—diets that favor pizza and fried chicken over fruits and vegetables, lifestyles that do little to encourage movement or activity—are nurtured and perpetuated in our homes and our communities. It makes sense, then, that our efforts in diabetes education and management should center on these places.

"A lot of health decisions are what we call social determinants, and education is necessary to turn those social determinants around," Dr. Albright says. "People spend a matter of hours in doctors' offices or hospitals, but they spend days, weeks, months, years in their homes, in their workplaces, in their schools, in their places of worship. So that's where we need to be working if we're going to beat diabetes."

There's Strength in Numbers

It's true that we don't yet know the root cause of diabetes, and we don't yet have a cure. Christopher Saudek, MD, a past president of the American Diabetes Association and director of the Johns Hopkins Comprehensive Diabetes Center in Baltimore, is among the experts who expect that we'll continue chipping away at these and other mysteries—though admittedly, any major breakthroughs may be years away. "We've seen some remarkable advances in the past 5 years, but some big questions remain," Dr. Saudek says. "So there has been good progress—just not the kind that comes across as a headline declaring, 'Diabetes Cured!'"

Until that day comes, we can use the knowledge and resources already at our disposal to stay a step ahead of diabetes. One of our objectives in creating this book for you is to put at your fingertips the information that will enable you to not just manage diabetes but truly master it. As you'll see, even modest lifestyle changes can dramatically improve your blood sugar control while protecting against complications.

Just as important, we want this book to make you feel part of a larger community of people—millions of them, in fact—who are thriving despite diabetes. Though the disease can seem isolating at times, it's important to remember that you're not on your own. The power of community is what's driving Dr. Albright and her colleagues to take the fight against diabetes to the streets. It's also one of the cornerstone principles of the American Association of Diabetes Educators (AADE), which designs programs to encourage those with diabetes to adopt a team approach in managing their care. "We want to tell the person with diabetes, 'You are not alone,'" says AADE president Amparo Gonzalez, RN. "You can't do it alone, and you don't have to."

The Many Faces of Diabetes

SO JUST WHAT IS DIABETES, anyway?

Simply put, diabetes occurs when your body is unable to properly process the glucose it gets from food. Glucose is a simple sugar that provides the necessary energy for cells to carry out their basic tasks. When this fuel can't get into cells, which is what happens in diabetes, they don't function as they should.

And what happens to all that glucose that isn't getting into cells, where it belongs? It stays in your bloodstream. The medical term for this is hyperglycemia. Having blood that's too rich in glucose is like having motor oil that's too thick for your car's engine: It mucks up the works. More precisely, it upsets the super-sensitive biochemical balances that enable the body to properly function, setting in motion a chain reaction of health problems, such as high cholesterol, high blood pressure, heart and kidney disease, and vision trouble.

All of this begs the question: Why can't your body use glucose as it should? It has to do with insulin, a hormone produced by the pancreas, an organ that is about the size of your hand and sits behind your stomach. Insulin serves a very specific purpose: It facilitates the body's use of glucose by escorting the sugar into cells. Cells won't let in just any substance; gaining entry requires a certain access code, which insulin has. Once it unlocks a cell, glucose can get inside.

At least, that's how it's supposed to work. There are two ways in which the partnership between insulin and glucose can break down: Either the pancreas stops making insulin, or the cells for some reason stop responding to insulin, which means glucose can't get in—a condition known as insulin resistance. In either case, there's a disruption of the energy supply to cells, with two results: The cells starve, and the blood becomes saturated with unused glucose. This combination of impoverished cells and too-rich blood is why the diabetic condition is sometimes described as starvation in the midst of plenty.

As this unhealthy blood courses through the body, it can set the stage for a host of complications. This is what makes diabetes such a serious and complex disease. An expert committee charged with defining diabetes for the American Diabetes Association (ADA) put it this way: "The chronic hyperglycemia of diabetes is associated with long-term damage, dysfunction, and failure of various organs, especially the eyes, kidneys, nerves, heart, and blood vessels."

We'll talk more about the widespread effects of diabetes in the next chapter, but the bottom line is clear: You must do what you can to keep this disease in check. To help you best accomplish that by being as informed as possible, let's delve a bit deeper into the various forms of the disease.

Type 1: A System Malfunction

The fundamental issue with type 1 diabetes is that the pancreas loses its ability to produce insulin. This happens because the body's immune system, for reasons not fully known, attacks the cells that produce insulin—they're called beta cells—and destroys them. People who develop type 1 diabetes realize rather quickly that something isn't quite right because the symptoms—lethargy or drowsiness, weight loss, excessive hunger and thirst, vision changes, labored breathing, and increased urination—tend to be sudden and severe.

Conventional medical wisdom long held that type 1 diabetes is an inherited condition, a view reinforced by the fact that type 1 is more common among whites than among other ethnic groups. But we now know that genes don't tell the whole story. One clue that genes aren't the only piece of the type 1 puzzle:

If one identical twin develops the disease, the odds are less than 50/50 that the other twin will, too.

The current thinking is that each person's risk of type 1 rises and falls with a combination of genetic and environmental factors, including diet and exposure to infection. In fact, researchers are looking much more closely at the role of environment. For the past 20 years, the number of people getting type 1 worldwide has been steadily increasing—and at a pace that can't be accounted for by genetics alone.

About half of those who have type 1 diabetes are diagnosed in childhood or their early teens, which is why for many years it was known as juvenile diabetes. That name has fallen out of favor, though, because we've learned that about 10 percent of those who are diagnosed with diabetes in adulthood have type 1. Often these people are initially misdiagnosed with type 2 because that's what doctors are accustomed to looking for in adults.

Type 2: A Production Shutdown

Of the two main forms of diabetes, type 2 is far more common, accounting for 90 to 95 percent of all cases. It differs from type 1 in that the pancreas does not stop producing insulin, at least not at the outset; rather, for reasons that still baffle scientists, the hormone simply stops working properly. As a result, the cells don't get the glucose that they need to do their jobs. (This is the insulin resistance that we discussed a bit earlier.) The net effect is the same for type 2 as for type 1: The cells are going hungry while the blood has glucose to spare.

Though in type 1 diabetes insulin production shuts down completely (which is why insulin injections are necessary), in type 2 the opposite occurs. The pancreas shifts into overdrive, pumping out even more insulin in an effort to get some of the glucose out of the bloodstream and into cells. It's a noble effort, but eventually—perhaps because the pancreas simply burns out—insulin production slows down, and the body's attempts to regulate its blood glucose levels are compromised even more.

Type 2 diabetes produces many of the same symptoms as type 1: fatigue, frequent urination, increased thirst and hunger, unexplained weight loss, blurred vision, and slow wound healing. The difference is that these symptoms tend to develop much more gradually—so gradually that you may have type 2 for years before you notice that something is wrong. The trouble is, the disease can do damage long before it's called out. One study, for example, revealed that diabetic retinopathy—a common complication that affects the blood vessels of the eyes—often begins at least 7 years before a clinical diagnosis of diabetes. This is just one way in which high blood glucose can cause trouble long before its symptoms become obvious.

As we discussed in the previous chapter, type 2 diabetes tends to favor those over age 50 who are overweight and out of shape, but just as type 1 diabetes is cropping up in adults, type 2 is affecting a growing number of children—rendering its alternative name, adult-onset diabetes, obsolete. Experts attribute this phenomenon to the escalating rate of obesity among 6- to 19-year-olds, which has almost tripled over the past 20 to 30 years. Just as in an adult, as a child's waistline expands, so does the risk of developing type 2 diabetes. "Think of youngsters with type 2 diabetes as the proverbial canaries in the coal mine," says Francine R. Kaufman, MD, a past president of the ADA and author of *Diabesity: The Obesity-Diabetes Epidemic That Threatens America—And What We Must Do to Stop It*. "They signal that something is very wrong and endangers us all."

One way in which obesity increases the risk of type 2 diabetes is by setting the stage for insulin resistance. There are a number of complex mechanisms by which this is thought to occur, not all of them fully understood. In essence, it's believed that fat cells, as a means of self-preservation, release chemicals into the blood that increase fat production. Because insulin's job is to turn glucose into energy, not fat, fat cells and insulin are, in a sense, natural enemies.

That said, not everyone with type 2 is overweight and out of shape. Many are—some 80 percent, according to one estimate—but for the rest, certain other factors must be at work. In fact, genetics may play an even stronger role in type 2 than in type 1. There's some evidence that the same genes responsible for predisposing people to diabetes may predispose them to obesity, too.

Genetics also helps explain why the incidence of type 2 diabetes is more prevalent among certain ethnic groups, including African Americans, Asian Americans, Hispanic Americans, and Native Americans. Still, we can't discount how lifestyle factors may be feeding into any genetic predisposition to diabetes. After all, the habits and behaviors that are passed down through generations—of eating certain traditional dishes, for example—may not be the healthiest for our waistlines or our diabetes risk.

"We Latinos love our food," says Amparo Gonzalez, RN, CDE, president of the American Association of Diabetes Educators (AADE) and director of the Georgia Latino Diabetes Program at Emory University School of Medicine in Atlanta. "Many of us fill our plates with tortillas and rice and beans and very few vegetables." But Latinos aren't the only ones with a penchant for certain dietary staples, Gonzalez adds. Every ethnic heritage has its traditional favorites. For Donna Rice, RN, who preceded Gonzalez as president of the AADE, it's pasta. "My family is Italian," she says. "If somebody handed me an eating plan that didn't include pasta three times a week, I wouldn't stick with it."

The point is, it's the combination of genes and lifestyle—not just one or the other—that's responsible for the surge in type 2 diabetes in the United States and around the world. This is why diabetes management almost always involves changes to help lose weight, exercise, eat better, and generally adopt a healthier lifestyle.

Prediabetes: The Early Warning System

Because the onset of type 2 diabetes tends to be so gradual, and because it can be doing damage all the while, doctors wanting to get an earlier jump on the disease are diagnosing what they've dubbed prediabetes. People with prediabetes have blood glucose levels that are higher than normal but not high enough to indicate diabetes. As many as 54 million American adults fall into this category, according to the National Institutes of Health.

TESTING FOR PREDIABETES

Finding out that your blood glucose level qualifies as prediabetic is like being on a drive and coming on a bank of flashing yellow lights and arrows pointing to a detour: The road's out ahead, and you'd best take evasive action to circumvent serious trouble.

To identify prediabetes as well as diabetes, doctors rely on two tests—one for fasting glucose, the other for glucose tolerance.

The fasting glucose test is just what it sounds like: You fast overnight, then get a blood test in the morning. A fasting blood glucose of 100 to 125 mg/dL (milligrams per deciliter of blood) is considered prediabetic. Your doctor may note this as IFG, which stands for "impaired fasting glucose." A reading of 126 mg/dL or higher, once confirmed by a second test, would qualify as diabetic.

A glucose tolerance test also requires fasting overnight. Your doctor will ask you to drink a sweet liquid to raise your blood glucose level. Then 2 hours later, you'll have a blood test to assess how well your body is processing the glucose. In the case of insulin resistance, the test will show a higher-than-normal level of glucose in the bloodstream, which means that the sugar hasn't been absorbed into your cells.

On a glucose tolerance test, a reading below 140 mg/dL is considered normal, while a reading between 140 and 199 mg/dL is prediabetic. Your doctor may label this with another set of initials—IGT, which stands for "impaired glucose tolerance." A reading above 200 mg/dL indicates full-blown diabetes.

A diagnosis of prediabetes is a sign that trouble's brewing. Chances are good that someone who's prediabetic will develop full-blown diabetes within 10 years unless he or she takes remedial action. The silver lining: It's possible to reverse—yes, *reverse*—prediabetes and head off type 2. On the other hand, allowing prediabetes to simmer can raise the risk of heart attack, stroke, and other cardiovascular problems—just like type 2. This is because high blood glucose, whether or not it reaches diabetic levels, can do damage anywhere in the body that blood flows—and that's everywhere.

METABOLIC SYNDROME: HIGH GLUCOSE AND MORE

Metabolic syndrome is a cluster of conditions, all of which could contribute to the development of both type 2 diabetes and cardiovascular disease. The conditions that fall under the metabolic syndrome label can vary according to who's defining it, but they usually include excess weight, especially around the waist (so-called visceral fat); high blood pressure; high LDL ("bad") cholesterol and triglycerides, along with low HDL ("good") cholesterol; and high blood glucose.

Not all doctors are sold on the idea of a metabolic syndrome. Some contend that attaching any name to such a constellation of conditions makes the metabolic syndrome seem like a condition unto itself (though even they might agree that's preferable to the original name, syndrome X, which seems more appropriate for a bad 1950s sci-fi movie).

Other doctors make the case that by grouping the various conditions under one label, it makes the point that the whole is much greater than the sum of its parts. In other words, having even one of the conditions of the metabolic syndrome spells trouble, but having three or more suggests a high risk of type 2 diabetes, heart disease—or both.

Doctors use two tests to detect both prediabetes and diabetes. One is a fasting glucose test; the other, a glucose tolerance test (see "Testing for Prediabetes" on page 19).

Gestational Diabetes: A Pregnancy Surprise

Somewhere between prediabetes, which is reversible, and diabetes, which is chronic, is gestational diabetes. As its name suggests, it comes and goes during pregnancy. Between 3 and 8 percent of women who are pregnant develop gestational diabetes.

Actually, it isn't unusual for a mom-to-be to experience a temporary case of insulin resistance. Studies have shown that women typically lose about 50 percent of their ability to process glucose during pregnancy. The pancreas responds by shifting into overdrive, increasing its insulin production by 200 percent or more.

The difference between "normal" levels of insulin resistance in pregnancy and gestational diabetes is one of degree. Doctors determine whether or not a woman has crossed that line by conducting blood glucose tests during pregnancy.

Gestational diabetes is thought to be a response to certain hormones that develop in the placenta around the 24th week of pregnancy. For example, a placental hormone called lactogen increases up to 30-fold, helping to ensure an adequate energy supply for the developing baby—and in the process, blocking insulin from doing its job.

As with other types of diabetes, certain lifestyle factors are likely to increase a woman's chances of developing gestational diabetes. For example, women who gain too much weight while pregnant may be at higher risk, as are those who are overweight or obese before conception. Then, too, some women become pregnant without realizing that they have type 2 diabetes, only to be diagnosed when they're tested for gestational diabetes. This is one reason that Richard Hellman, MD, president of the American Association of Clinical Endocrinologists and clinical professor of medicine at the University of Missouri Kansas City School of Medicine, advocates diabetes testing for all moms-to-be on the first obstetric visit rather than waiting until later in pregnancy, as is often the case. Babies born to women with type 1 or type 2 diabetes are at greater risk for birth defects, including malformations of the brain, heart, and spine. So the sooner the mom begins treatment, Dr. Hellman says, the healthier the baby will be.

Gestational diabetes generally doesn't cause such serious complications, but it does pose risks. In particular, the glucose in the mother's blood creates a diet that's much too rich for the baby. This can lead to what doctors call macrosomia, a technical term for what amounts to baby fat. If the baby gets too big, it

BREASTFEEDING: NATURAL BLOOD GLUCOSE CONTROL FOR NEW MOMS

The potential health effects of gestational diabetes on a developing baby may leave a new mom wondering whether her high blood glucose could prevent her from breastfeeding. In fact, compelling research suggests that breastfeeding may be one of the healthiest things that she can do—not just for her baby but for herself, too.

Doctors long have known that as a woman's metabolic systems return to normal after childbirth, her insulin resistance drops by 50 to 70 percent and her blood glucose begins to stabilize. According to a study published in the *Journal of the American Medical Association,* breastfeeding actually enhances this process by helping to balance blood glucose. The study also found that women who breastfeed longer are less likely to develop type 2 diabetes later in life—perhaps in part by facilitating postpartum weight loss, as the study's authors speculate. This protective effect did not extend to women with gestational diabetes, however.

Actually, new moms who are breastfeeding—even those who had gestational diabetes during pregnancy—need to pay attention that their blood glucose levels don't drop too low (a condition known as hypoglycemia). That's because breastfeeding typically drains some 900 calories a day from the mother's system, unless she eats more to make up for them.

For new moms who've been diagnosed with type 1 or type 2 diabetes, the steeper fluctuations in blood glucose levels that come with breastfeeding must be watched carefully. Smaller, more frequent meals, along with more frequent blood sugar checks, help offset the peaks and valleys in blood glucose levels. As long as appropriate precautions are taken, says Richard Hellman, MD, immediate past president of the American Association of Clinical Endocrinologists and clinical professor of medicine at the University of Missouri Kansas City School of Medicine, "we think that breastfeeding is healthier for both mother and child, and we encourage it."

can make for a more difficult delivery, including a greater likelihood of Caesarean section. What's more, as babies born to women with gestational diabetes grow up, they're more likely to develop type 2 diabetes.

Maintaining good blood glucose control during pregnancy can greatly reduce the risks of gestational diabetes for both the mother and her baby. And the good news is, the condition goes away once baby is born. Women who develop gestational diabetes during one pregnancy, though, are twice as likely to get it during subsequent pregnancies. They also become much more likely to develop type 2 diabetes within 15 years.

What's In a Name?

When diagnosing patients with diabetes, doctors usually identify the disease according to the types we've described here. Interestingly, though, current research suggests that diabetes may not be so easily categorized. A 2003 report by the ADA's Expert Committee on the Diagnosis and Classification of Diabetes Mellitus described diabetes as a "clinically heterogeneous [dissimilar] group of disorders" that share one particular feature: hyperglycemia, or high blood sugar. The report goes on to say that "assigning a type of diabetes to an individual often depends on the circumstances present at the time of diagnosis, and many diabetic individuals do not easily fit into a single class."

What all this means is that each of us has the potential to develop a unique version of diabetes, based on a combination of genetic makeup, physical condition at various life stages, exposure to specific environments, and life experiences. Given all of these variables, the number of potential manifestations of the disease downright boggles the mind. "We already know that there are at least dozens if not hundreds of 'flavors' of diabetes, and there could be thousands," says John Buse, MD, PhD, president of medicine and science for the ADA. "For purposes of clinical convenience, we've lumped them into categories like type 1 and type 2, but there are many, many more types than that."

Dr. Buse adds that the broad categories of type 1 and type 2 do comfortably accommodate the vast majority of people with diabetes, which can be helpful especially for determining a course of treatment. But as our knowledge base about the many faces of the disease grows, so will our ability to effectively control it. As Dr. Buse explains, "When we eventually enter an era of molecular medicine, we'll be able to identify exactly what genes aren't working properly, and—theoretically—we'll have treatments to address each of those genetic defects more precisely."

One of the primary objectives of current diabetes research is to find the most elemental cause or causes that set the stage for the disease. Here, too, there are numerous factors at play, but scientists are looking for larger commonalities. In other words, if diabetes is a progressive disease, what gets the ball rolling? Here again, Dr. Buse says, scientists have hundreds of hypotheses but no definitive answers—yet. "It's a little bit like asking, what is the meaning of life? It's almost unknowable," he explains. "It's like taking a photo of something. We can see what's in the frame, but it's what we can't see that might be very important."

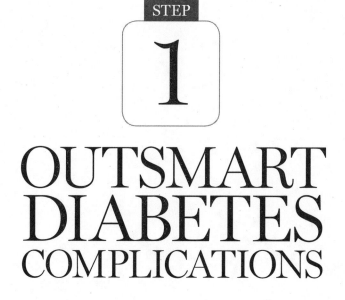

OUTSMART DIABETES COMPLICATIONS

Vision Problems (Retinopathy)

IF YOU HAVE DIABETES, you'll want to do everything possible to steer yourself clear of eye problems, a major complication of the disease. Diabetes steals the sight of 12,000 to 24,000 people each year and is responsible for 8 percent of blindness in the United States, making it the leading cause of new blindness in people ages 20 to 74, according to the American Diabetes Association.

One problem even reflects in its name the close relationship between diabetes and the eyes: diabetic retinopathy, a catchall term that refers to diabetes-related damage to the retina. This is the nerve layer that lines the back of the eye, senses light, and creates impulses that reach the brain through the optic nerve. The damage causes progressive eye disease that may start with no symptoms at all and end with no sight at all—unless you're diligent about managing your diabetes and wise about seeking proper care for your eyes.

Though our focus is on diabetic retinopathy, people with diabetes also have a higher risk of other eye problems, including cataracts (clouding of the lens), glaucoma (increased pressure inside the eye), and a variety of common diseases that affect the cornea.

What's the Connection?

Scientists don't yet understand how diabetes causes retinopathy, but they know high blood glucose is the key factor. Over time, increased blood glucose can inflame and weaken the tiny blood vessels in the eyes, slowing blood flow and depriving the retina of oxygen. In response to this damage, the body secretes a protein called vascular endothelial growth factor (VEGF), which promotes the growth of new blood vessels in the eye. But they may grow in the wrong place, damaging the eye and causing partial or full blindness.

The most common form of diabetic retinopathy is called nonproliferative retinopathy. When you have this condition, the blood vessels that feed your retina develop weak spots that bulge, swell, and leak fluid into surrounding tissue. The disease may not progress past the mildest stage and may not require treatment—or it may become moderate to severe, with the blood vessels becoming increasingly blocked. Even at this stage, you may have no symptoms or loss of vision.

In some people, nonproliferative retinopathy eventually progresses to the more serious form, proliferative retinopathy, in which the blood vessels close off. In response, fragile new blood vessels grow on the retina and into the back of the eye (a process called neovascularization). These abnormal blood vessels often rupture and bleed in what is known as a vitreous hemorrhage, causing blurred vision or temporary blindness. Or, again, you may have no symptoms at all.

Retinal detachment, a more advanced stage, produces scar tissue that grows and peels the retina away from the back of the eye. At first, the detachment may be slight; but if you don't get immediate treatment, the whole retina may detach, leading to severe vision loss or blindness.

At any stage of the disease, you may also experience macular edema, where fluid accumulates around the macula. The macula sits near the sensitive center of the retina at the back of your eyeball, so any swelling in this area may blur your central vision.

Diabetic retinopathy can affect other parts of the eye as well. Whether or not you experience early vision symptoms, the longer you have diabetes, the more likely you are to have retinopathy. If you keep your blood sugar levels tightly controlled and close to normal, you'll be less likely to develop this condition—or at least you'll have to deal only with the milder form.

How Common Is It?

Diabetic retinopathy is the most common complication of type 2 diabetes, currently affecting more than 4.1 million Americans age 40 and older. Up to 21 percent of people with type 2 diabetes already have diabetic retinopathy by the time they're diagnosed with diabetes. Almost 100 percent of people with type 1 and more than 70 percent with type 2 diabetes eventually develop diabetic retinopathy, in most cases without vision loss, according to a Johns Hopkins University special report. Nearly 900,000 Americans currently have diabetic retinopathy severe enough to cause vision loss.

Mexican Americans are almost twice as likely to develop diabetic retinopathy, and non-Hispanic blacks are almost 50 percent as likely to develop this condition as non-Hispanic whites.

What Is My Risk?

If you have type 1 or type 2 diabetes, you know you are already at risk for diabetic retinopathy. The longer you have diabetes, the more likely you are to develop it. To find out what other risk factors may threaten your vision, answer these questions.

1. Do you have diabetes and are not successfully managing your blood sugar levels?

2. Do you have high blood pressure and have trouble keeping it under control?

3. Do you have high LDL ("bad") cholesterol and triglycerides?

4. Is your heritage Hispanic or African American?

5. Is your vision blurry?

6. Do you have trouble reading signs or books?

7. Do you sometimes see double?

8. Do you have pain in one or both eyes?

9. Are your eyes usually red?

10. Do you feel pressure in one or both eyes?

11. Do you see spots or floaters?

12. Do straight lines not look straight to you?

13. Do you have trouble seeing things off to the side like you used to?

The more yes answers you have to questions 1 through 4, the more your risk increases. If you answered yes to any of questions 5 through 13, you may have undiagnosed symptoms of the disease. See your eye care specialist for an evaluation.

What Should I Watch For?

For people with type 1 diabetes, mild damage to the retina begins about 7 years after the onset of diabetes, but vision changes don't usually develop until years later.

If you've recently been diagnosed with type 2 diabetes, you may already have retinopathy without knowing it, or you may soon develop it. By the time you realize you have diabetes, dangerous changes in the retina may have occurred, but your vision may seem fine as long as you're in the early (nonproliferative retinopathy) stage.

Once the disease progresses to the proliferative retinopathy stage, bleeding in the eye may cause blurred vision, or you may see spots, flashing lights, or floaters. You may lose vision toward the side (peripheral vision) or experience rapid severe or complete vision loss.

If the retina becomes detached, your vision may be wavy or watery. A dark shadow may appear in your side (peripheral) vision, or you may experience sudden blindness in one eye. At any stage of diabetic retinopathy, your vision may be severely blurred by fluid accumulating around the macula (that's macular edema). You may also feel pain or pressure in one or both eyes.

What Can I Do about It?

In a study of 11,247 women and men, researchers from the International Diabetes Institute in Australia compared the results from A1C testing, which gives a picture of average glucose control over the past 2 to 3 months. They found that the odds for retinopathy rose 25 percent when A1C levels were more than 7.5 percent for up to 4 years and rose 50 percent when A1C remained high for more than 8 years. For most people in the study, the onset of diabetic retinopathy coincided with the time their diabetes was diagnosed. The researchers say annual screening for diabetic retinopathy and managing

 When to See the Doctor

For people with type 1 diabetes, the American Academy of Ophthalmology recommends yearly screening beginning 5 years after diagnosis. For type 2, see your ophthalmologist annually for a dilated eye exam. If found early and monitored, both proliferative retinopathy and macular edema can be treated.

See your doctor if you see spots or floaters, have eye pain, pressure in one or both eyes, blurred or double vision, peripheral vision loss, trouble seeing straight lines, or chronically red eyes. Also ask your doctor to check for signs of cataracts and glaucoma.

Retinal detachment is a medical emergency that requires urgent medical care.

diabetes risk factors will help reduce the possibility of blindness caused by the disease. The following are some of the best sight-saving strategies.

Lifestyle Measures

■ **MANAGE YOUR BLOOD SUGAR.** Keep your blood sugar as close to normal as possible to minimize damage from retinopathy and slow its progression. According to a Centers for Disease Control and Prevention survey of 15,000 people with diabetes, fewer than 45 percent checked their blood sugar levels daily. Without treatment and adequate blood sugar control, diabetic retinopathy usually gets worse.

■ **GET YOUR VISION CORRECTED.** People with diabetes who also have vision problems often don't realize their sight will improve with the proper prescription for glasses or contact lenses, according to the CDC research. In the survey, 11 percent of people with diabetes had 20/40 visual acuity or worse in their best eye. (Normal is 20/20.) But 65 percent of those surveyed still didn't have their vision corrected with an accurate prescription.

■ **WATCH YOUR BLOOD PRESSURE.** Lowering your blood pressure could save your eyesight, say British scientists. When they compared 758 people with diabetes who strictly controlled their blood pressure (keeping it around 144/82 mm Hg) with those whose levels stayed higher (157/88), the better-controlled group had a 47 percent lower risk of dimmed eyesight. High blood pressure can damage blood vessels in the eyes, explains study author David Matthews, FRCP, chairman of the Oxford Centre for Diabetes, Endocrinology, and Metabolism. Keep your blood pressure at healthy levels with exercise; weight loss; plenty of fruits, veggies, and whole grains; and, if needed, medication.

■ **GO FISHIN' FOR BETTER VISION.** A new major study of mice found that the omega-3 fatty acids in fish protect against the development and progression of retinopathy. In the journal *Nature Medicine*, the researchers reported that upping omega-3 fatty acids and cutting omega-6 fatty acids (the most common type in the standard American diet) reduced the area of vessel loss that leads to abnormal blood vessel growth and blindness.

A higher amount of omega-6s contributed to the growth of abnormal blood vessels in the retina. But just a 2 percent bump in dietary omega-3 intake eased the severity of retinopathy by 40 to 50 percent. The promising results may have something to do with the unusually high concentrations of omega-3 fatty acids in the retina, reports lead author Kip M. Connor, PhD, a postdoctoral research fellow at Children's Hospital Boston, an affiliate of Harvard Medical School. To get more omega-3s in your diet, go for fatty fish like mackerel, lake trout, herring, sardines, albacore tuna, and salmon.

■ **EAT A BOWL OF BLUEBERRIES.** Antioxidants called anthocyanins in red and purple berries may help reduce eye damage from the sun and normal aging, as well as boost healthy blood flow to your eyes. Studies show that these plant pigments may also slow the development of diabetic retinopathy by strengthening blood vessel walls. Along with blueberries, fill up on anthocyanin-rich cherries, red grapes (also grape juice and red wine), and pomegranates.

■ **MUNCH ON NUTS.** A 5-year Harvard Medical School study found that eating nuts at least once a week slowed vision deterioration by 40 percent. Experts suspect the healthy fat in nuts may prevent excess total fat from clogging the arteries in your eyes, just as it protects the arteries in your heart.

■ **CHILL OUT.** Staying relaxed and calm may help bring down your blood

If you're planning to have surgery to treat cataracts, be warned: It may actually worsen diabetic retinopathy.

British researchers looked at the retinas of diabetic patients before and after cataract surgery using orange dye and a camera to take pictures (fluorescein angiography). Diabetic retinopathy worsened in four out of six patients. The researchers also found a large increase in two factors that boost troublesome blood vessel growth: vascular endothelial growth factor (VEGF) and hepatocyte growth factor (HGF).

The surgery also decreased one of the good factors—pigment epithelium derived factor (PEDF), which works to prevent formation of these damaging new blood vessels—and increased an inflammatory chemical messenger called interleukin 1B. While this is typical after surgery, it can also trigger VEGF and HGF.

Researchers are currently investigating new treatments for diabetic retinopathy that may control these growth factor levels post-op. One possibility is a prescription eye drop called nepafenac ophthalmic, a non-steroidal anti-inflammatory drug typically used after cataract surgery. An animal study published in the February 2007 journal *Diabetes* reports that the drops may help reduce retinal microvascular problems and other eye abnormalities.

sugar levels and, consequently, lower your risk of complications such as diabetic retinopathy and blindness, according to research from the Medical University of Ohio. In the 10-week study of 30 people, 15 practiced daily tension-taming exercises, such as muscle relaxation, and had their techniques monitored with weekly 45-minute biofeedback sessions. The other 15 took diabetes education classes.

At the end of the study, those who learned to chill out saw about a 10 percent drop in fasting blood sugar and in the level of A1C. "Stress triggers hormones that raise blood sugar," explains lead researcher Ronald McGinnis, MD. "Reducing chronic stress switches this process off." If that's not motivation enough, the relaxation group also experienced a drop in depression and anxiety. To find a biofeedback therapist, check out the Web site of the Biofeedback Certification Institute of America (bcia.org) and click on Find a Practitioner.

Medical Treatments

■ **LASER THERAPY.** Several types of laser therapy are used to treat diabetic retinopathy. Photocoagulation, the most common treatment, makes tiny laser burns on the retina to seal leaky blood vessels and stop their growth. Scatter photocoagulation (also known as panretinal photocoagulation) creates hundreds of tiny laser burns in one or two treatments. It's also useful in some cases of glaucoma. Focal photocoagulation aims the laser directly at a leaking blood vessel in the macula.

■ **VITRECTOMY.** Your doctor may recommend this eye surgery when laser therapy is no longer effective in treating your retinopathy. Vitrectomy removes scar tissue, blood, and part or all of the vitreous (the jellylike fluid that fills the eyeball) and replaces it with a clear liquid. A surgeon may also use this technique to reattach the retina, but the success rate for reattachment is only about 50 percent.

Gum Disease

WHEN YOU THINK ABOUT GUM DISEASE, the heart—much less diabetes—may not be the first thing that comes to mind. But in the big picture of diabetes—a place where every condition and complication seems to be connected to the next—experts say that oral health is most certainly intertwined with blood sugar control and circulation issues.

What's the Connection?

Diabetes hits your gums with a triple whammy. First: "The thickening of blood vessels is a complication of diabetes that may increase risk for gum disease," says Mark J. Escoto, DDS, founder of the Nevada TMJ Institute in Las Vegas. "Blood vessels deliver oxygen and nourishment to the body tissues, including the mouth, and carry away the waste products. Diabetes slows the flow of nutrients and removal of wastes, which can weaken the resistance of gum and bone tissue to infection."

Second: Diabetes increases sugar levels not only in the blood, leading to thickened vessels, but in the saliva as well. And more sugar in the mouth provides a fertile breeding ground for bacteria and other germs that cause infection and lead to gum disease. "In uncontrolled diabetes, the higher levels of glucose in the mouth's fluids may help germs grow and set the stage for gum disease," says Dr. Escoto.

A third strike against your gums: "People with diabetes are at a higher risk for infections in general," says Rajesh V. Lalla, BDS, PhD, assistant professor of oral medicine at the University of Connecticut Health Center in Farmington. "Periodontal disease is inflammation of the gums and bone surrounding teeth due to uncontrolled infection." So combine high sugar in the blood and saliva with decreased immune function, and it's clear why gum disease risk runs so high in people with diabetes.

That's not to say you're destined for gum disease. The key to keeping your mouth healthy is keeping your blood sugar at bay. "Gum disease is linked to diabetic control," says Dr. Escoto. "People with poor blood sugar control tend to get gum disease more often and more severely, and they lose more teeth than those with good control."

In fact, beyond being a complication of diabetes, gum disease can also be a warning sign, says Dr. Lalla: "Periodontal disease may develop in the pre-diabetic stage and arouse suspicion of diabetes, especially if present in combination with other common signs and symptoms of diabetes, such as increased thirst and increased urination."

How Common Is It?

According to Dr. Lalla, people with poor control of their blood sugar appear to run a much greater risk of gum disease than those who keep their diabetes under control. "An analysis of data from more than 4,000 subjects demonstrated that patients with poorly controlled diabetes had a highly significant 2.9-fold increased risk for severe periodontal disease than those without diabetes," he says. "On the other hand, well-controlled diabetics did not have a statistically significant increase in risk."

Not only are those with poorly controlled diabetes more likely to get gum disease, but their gum problems will likely be much worse. "Periodontal disease is more prevalent, progresses more rapidly, and is often more severe in individuals with both type 1 and type 2 diabetes," says JoAnn R. Gurenlian, PhD, chair of the Pharmacy, Podiatry, Optometry, and Dental Professionals' (PPOD) Work Group of the National Diabetes Education Program. "However, if individuals partner with a dentist and dental hygienist, have regular examinations and professional treatment, and perform daily preventive home care, they can control the oral effects of the disease."

What Is My Risk?

The good news about gum disease: Compared with other diabetes complications, it's much more preventable. The first step toward saving your teeth is assessing your symptoms and evaluating your risk. These questions from our experts will help you figure it out.

- Do you have problems controlling your blood sugar?

- Do you brush and floss less than twice a day?

- Do you have your teeth cleaned professionally less than twice a year?

- Do you drink alcohol or smoke?

- Do your gums bleed when you brush or floss or at any other time?

- Are your gums red, swollen, or tender?

- Do you often have bad breath or a bad taste in your mouth?

- Have you noticed any loose teeth, changes in the way they fit together, or shift in the way any dental apparatuses fit?

Determining your risk of gum disease is fairly straightforward: The more you answered yes, the greater your risk.

What Should I Watch For?

Nobody wants gum disease. But if there's a silver lining to this plight, it's that the signs are easy to recognize and act upon.

If you have diabetes and gum disease, the best-case scenario is to catch it at the first sign. But even if symptoms progress, you can still take measures to preserve your mouth's health. In addition, Dr. Gurenlian says, a few symptoms are more prevalent among people with diabetes. Here's how gum disease tends to play itself out.

EARLY-STAGE SYMPTOMS

- Dry mouth
- Gums that bleed during brushing, flossing, or eating
- Bad breath
- Early signs of tooth decay

ADVANCED-STAGE SYMPTOMS

- Gums appear to pull away from teeth
- Red, tender, or swollen gums
- Pus between teeth and gums
- Chronic bad taste in the mouth
- Loose teeth
- Change in the way your teeth fit together or a dental apparatus fits
- Visible tooth decay or cavities

SYMPTOMS UNIQUE TO PEOPLE WITH DIABETES

- Breath that smells fruity or like acetone
- Candidiasis (a fungal infection)
- Increased incidence of dental abscesses (swollen, pus-filled sores)
- Burning sensation
- Slick, viscous saliva
- Swollen parotid gland, which is the largest salivary gland; this must be diagnosed by your doctor

What Can I Do about It?

If you have diabetes, fighting gum disease is a two-pronged attack: treating the diabetes symptoms themselves and stepping up your oral hygiene. Consider the steps below your action plan for preventing diabetes-related gum disease, as well as keeping symptoms at bay.

■ **GET YOUR BLOOD SUGAR UNDER CONTROL.** We've already established the strong tie between managing blood sugar and preventing gum disease, but Dr. Gurenlian says the relationship is more intricate than most people realize. "Research has shown that having good glucose control will help improve oral health," she says. "Conversely, having good oral health improves glucose control. It's a two-way relationship." In a Spanish study of 20 people with gum disease, researchers found that the patients' blood sugar dropped by as much as 20 percent and stayed there for 3 months after they received treatment for gum disease.

In addition to the oral health tips below, the best ways to control your blood sugar are to check it regularly for fluctuations and eat a sound diet. Ideally, you'll work with a dietitian to develop an individualized nutrition plan. "A customized diet for anyone, but especially for someone with diabetes, should be tailored to size, activity level, lifestyle, preferences, medications, medical history, culture, and the socioeconomic status of the individual," says Bernadette Latson, RD, assistant professor of clinical nutrition at the University of Texas Southwestern Medical Center at Dallas.

■ **GIVE YOURSELF AN ORAL EXAM.** Considering the increased risk of diabetes—coupled with the fact that diabetes-related gum disease often doesn't present any pain—Dr. Gurenlian encourages her patients to conduct monthly mouth self-exams. You can do it in front of a mirror, looking for the signs and symptoms listed above.

■ **STEP UP YOUR ORAL CARE.** One of the easiest ways to fight the increased risk of gum disease, says Dr. Escoto, is by increasing your oral care accordingly. This includes brushing three or more times a day and flossing every night. Dr. Escoto also recommends investing in an electric toothbrush, which may do a more thorough job of cleaning teeth.

■ **DON'T AGGRAVATE DRY MOUTH.** One easily overlooked risk factor and warning sign of gum disease is dry mouth. And most mouthwashes contain alcohol, which further dries the mouth, says Harold Katz, DDS, author of *The Bad Breath Bible* and founder of California Breath Clinics. A better choice is

---

RESEARCH BUZZ

Faster, Easier Treatment for Gum Disease

Though the risk of gum disease remains high for people with diabetes, doctors continue to make great strides in treating periodontitis, says Mark J. Escoto, DDS, founder of the Nevada TMJ Institute in Las Vegas. For example, using lasers along with standard dental tools for scaling and root planing seems to improve the effectiveness of the procedure.

Meanwhile, two new prescription medications, Periostat and Atridox, have greatly sped up the healing process. "Periostat aids in healing by blocking the enzymes that break down soft tissue," Dr. Escoto says. "Atridox places the medicine directly into the soft tissue and releases antibiotics for up to 28 days, which helps get rid of the infection."

an alcohol-free mouthwash, says Dr. Katz, who sells two kinds—TheraBreath and PerioTherapy. Companies such as Crest, Oral-B, and Biotene also make alcohol-free mouthwashes.

■ **FIND A FROTH-FREE TOOTHPASTE.** Though the concerns about sodium lauryl sulfate (SLS), the foaming agent in most toothpastes and shampoos, have been largely overblown, Dr. Katz says, there is some evidence that abscesses and other wounds in the mouth may heal faster when patients use SLS-free toothpaste. Several companies, including Tom's of Maine, make these products.

■ **MAKE AN EXTRA DATE WITH YOUR DENTIST.** Brushing and flossing aren't the only habits that should become more frequent, says Dr. Escoto. You should also ask your dentist if more frequent visits are appropriate. "Depending on the severity or progression of the disease, you might need up to four cleanings a year, as well as deep cleanings, such as scaling and root planing," he says. These procedures remove plaque and tartar below the gum line in periodontal patients.

■ **GIVE UP CIGARETTES AND ALCOHOLIC DRINKS.** Smoking can inhibit blood flow, which may mask some of the more serious warning signs and symptoms of gum disease. And both smoking and drinking alcohol dry out your mouth, which eliminates the protective effects of saliva and puts you at even greater risk for developing gum disease.

■ **TRY VITAMIN C.** Among its other health benefits, Dr. Katz says, vitamin C is well known for its ability to repair and strengthen tissues throughout the body, including the gums. The recommended daily intake of vitamin C is 65 milligrams, easily obtained from a multivitamin or an orange.

■ **CHOOSE Q10.** Dr. Katz adds coenzyme Q10 to his list of supplements that strengthen the gums. Dosages range from 30 to 300 milligrams a day in three divided doses, so it's best to ask your doctor what amount might be right for you. In addition, Dr. Katz sells gel toothpaste called PerioTherapy that contains coenzyme Q10 for topical application to the gums.

■ **STICK TO OTHER DIABETES DOS.** Of course, all of these oral health–specific approaches don't lessen the importance of diabetes basics. Losing

The Diabetes Lowdown

If you have diabetes and gum disease, prepare to spend more time in the dentist's chair. Though it exhibits many of the same symptoms as regular gum disease, a diabetes-related case can be more complicated to treat, says JoAnn R. Gurenlian, PhD, chair of the Pharmacy, Podiatry, Optometry, and Dental Professionals (PPOD) Work Group of the National Diabetes Education Program. Expect longer dental appointments, including an in-depth conversation with your oral health professional. "Patients should be prepared to update their medical history at each appointment and pro-vide specific information concerning the medicines they are taking and how often they experience hypo-glycemia," says Dr. Gurenlian.

Come equipped with more than info. Bring your glucometer to dental appointments, and check your blood glucose reading in the office. "Having this information readily available allows dental professionals to provide more complete care and avoid the risk of a hypoglycemic emergency," says Dr. Gurenlian. If the appointment is scheduled to last longer than an hour, she suggests packing a small, healthy snack.

weight, lowering cholesterol, reducing blood pressure, eating a sound diet, and exercising regularly are vital to preventing spikes in blood sugar that lead to gum disease. Jackie Keller, a nutritionist and founding director of Nutri-Fit, a nutritional services and health education company, suggests focusing on mini meals to regulate blood sugar. "I tell my clients to eat five or six smaller, balanced meals, spaced evenly every 2 to 3 hours, throughout the day," she says. "In addition, try to eat at the same time each day. A regular schedule is important."

Heart Disease

OF ALL THE RISKS faced by people with diabetes or prediabetes, none is more serious than the danger posed by heart disease. Granted, heart disease is a concern for almost everyone: It's the number one killer of both men and women in America, claiming almost 900,000 lives or responsible for 36 percent of all deaths in 2004. People with diabetes are at an even greater risk—but if you're taking steps to control diabetes, you're automatically practicing some heart-healthy habits, too.

What's the Connection?

When it comes to why those with diabetes are at greater risk of developing heart disease, things get a little complicated. Researchers still don't have all the pieces of the intricate puzzle that is heart disease and diabetes. What they do know is that diabetes presents several risk factors, both direct and indirect, that multiply the chances of developing heart disease.

One of the most crucial direct risk factors is insulin resistance, which is the main symptom of type 2 diabetes. "Insulin resistance affects the central nervous system, causing high blood pressure, which in turn leads to heart disease," says David L. Katz, MD, MPH, director of the Yale Prevention Research Center in Derby, Connecticut, and author of *The Way to Eat.* "In addition, a diabetic's higher blood glucose levels can cause glycosylation, in which the glucose actually sticks to blood cells and contributes to clogged arteries."

Number one on the list of indirect risk factors: obesity. Excess weight leads to type 2 diabetes, but it also contributes to other risk factors for heart disease, including high blood pressure and high cholesterol. "According to the Centers for Disease Control and Prevention, two out of five people with diabetes do not have good control of their cholesterol, and one out of three does not have good blood pressure control," says Beverly Caskey, RPh, a Medco pharmacist who specializes in diabetes care. "Although most diabetic patients may be aware that heart disease is a complication of diabetes, they may not realize that by keeping cholesterol and blood pressure under control, they can significantly reduce, delay, or even prevent heart problems."

How Common Is It?

Add it all up, and it's not surprising to learn that people with diabetes are at greater risk for developing heart disease than the population at large. "Compared with the general population, diabetics are about seven times more likely to have heart failure, five times more likely to have a heart attack, and four times more likely to have coronary artery disease," says Caskey. What's more, people with diabetes are two to three times more likely to die as a result of a heart-related problem.

Other research has shown that people with diabetes have the same risk of a heart attack as diabetes-free people who've already had one. "From 1994 to 2004, the death rate from coronary heart disease declined 33 percent in the general population," says Judith Stanton, MD, an instructor in the internal medicine residency program at Alameda County Medical Center in California. "However, it is estimated that more than 65 percent of diabetic adults still die of heart disease or stroke."

What Is My Risk?

Having diabetes increases virtually all cardiovascular risk factors, whether it's heart disease or a heart attack, but the news isn't all bad. "The strategies for managing your risk of heart disease as a diabetic are virtually the same as in the population at large," says Dr. Katz. "You'll just want to take the advice very seriously!"

Those strategies include everything from managing your blood sugar to maintaining a proper diet, exercising, losing weight, quitting smoking, and keeping blood pressure and blood cholesterol levels under control. "Blood pressure control reduces the risk for heart disease and stroke among people with diabetes by 33 to 50 percent," says Dr. Stanton. "Improved control of blood cholesterol levels can reduce cardiovascular complications by 20 to 50 percent."

Having diabetes or prediabetes isn't the only factor to consider. The following questions will help you further determine your risk of developing heart disease.

- Do you have a family history of heart disease?

- Do you smoke?

- Is your BMI (body mass index) greater than 25?

- Is your waistline greater than 34 inches (if you're a woman) or 40 inches (if you're a man)?

- Is your total cholesterol greater than 200 mg/dL (milligrams per deciliter)?

- Is your blood triglyceride level higher than 150 mg/dL?

- Is your blood pressure 140/90 mm Hg (millimeters of mercury) or higher?

- Would you describe yourself as inactive?

- Have you previously had a heart attack or stroke?

Those nine questions cover the American Heart Association's risk factors for coronary heart disease, as well as a few extras thrown in by our experts. The more yes answers to the questions, the higher your risk. For the questions that involve numbers, higher numbers in your answers equal increased risk. For example, a person with a total cholesterol level of more than 300 is at higher risk than someone with a level of 240.

What Should I Watch For?

Considering the high stakes of heart disease or a heart attack, the primary objective of treatment is working with your doctor to prevent symptoms before they start. "The main point here is that a lot of heart disease is asymptomatic, and sometimes the first symptom you experience can be a fatal heart attack," says Elizabeth Barrett-Connor, MD, professor and chair of the department of family and preventive medicine at the University of California, San Diego. "That's why prevention is so important."

People with diabetes, who are at even greater risk, need to be even more vigilant about treatment. "Diabetics can have silent heart disease or silent heart attacks, with no chest pain at all," says Dr. Stanton. "Therefore, it is of

When to See the Doctor

- If you are overweight or inactive; have high blood cholesterol, high blood pressure, or a family history of heart disease; smoke; or previously experienced a heart attack or stroke, you need to be under a doctor's supervision for diabetes and heart disease risk.

- If you already have diabetes or prediabetes, you should see your doctor for regular physical exams, as well as screening tests for high blood pressure, high cholesterol, kidney disease, and other risk factors for heart disease.

- If you experience shortness of breath, fatigue, fainting, dizziness, heart palpitations, chest heaviness or tightness, or pain or tightness in your neck, jaw, shoulder, or arm, seek emergency medical attention immediately.

utmost importance to see your doctor regularly for screening tests. Even if you don't have any symptoms, you need regular physical exams and blood and urine tests to screen for high blood pressure, high cholesterol, and kidney disease, all of which are silent until they have caused irreversible damage."

Though most cases of heart disease don't present any symptoms until some damage has already been done, your body may provide you with some warning signs telling you to seek help immediately. These include:

- Shortness of breath
- Fatigue or fainting
- Dizziness
- Chest heaviness or tightness
- Neck, jaw, shoulder, or arm pain or tingling
- Heart palpitations

If you notice these or any other unusual or out-of-the-ordinary symptoms, see your doctor as soon as possible because they might be signs of heart disease or even a heart attack. People with diabetes especially need to be in tune with their symptoms because they might otherwise be more likely to ignore them. "Although the signs and symptoms of heart problems are the same for people with diabetes and the general population, diabetics may dismiss some of the symptoms, such as fatigue or fainting, thinking they are caused by low blood sugar," says Caskey. "Also, they may think that shortness of breath or heart palpitations are from being out of shape and may not seek medical help for early intervention."

What Can I Do about It?

When it comes to handling diabetes and heart disease, the recommendations aren't much different than what they are for the general population—but extra diligence is in order. "The advice on preventing heart disease for those with diabetes is the same as for those who have previously had a heart attack," says Dr. Katz. "That gives you a sense of how seriously the health community takes this risk."

Luckily, managing heart disease doesn't really complicate life for someone with diabetes, as the steps for managing the two conditions often overlap. "The things that improve diabetes are the same things that decrease your risk of heart disease," says Dr. Stanton. Here's what can help.

■ **MANAGE YOUR BLOOD SUGAR.** When you look at the connection between high blood sugar and heart disease, it's easy to understand why our experts cite this as the number one way to reduce your risk of heart disease. "High blood sugar plays a direct role in the development of atherosclerosis," says Dr. Stanton. "Multiple studies have shown that higher blood sugar levels lead to more oxidative damage to the blood vessels that supply the heart."

■ **GET TO KNOW THE GLYCEMIC INDEX.** In some cases, medication may be necessary to bring blood sugar under control. However, says Dr. Stanton, "diet is the most important factor in glycemic control." And nutritionists have developed a powerful tool to help you in this quest—the glycemic index. In the most basic terms, the glycemic index ranks foods by the impact they have on your blood glucose levels. The foods that affect blood sugar the least are some of the smartest choices for keeping diabetes symptoms under control.

RESEARCH BUZZ ....

The Inflammation Connection

Another growing area in diabetes and heart disease research is inflammation's contribution to both. Inflammation's not all bad: It's a sign that your body has sent out white blood cells and other infection-fighting chemicals to protect you from harm. But sometimes the release is misdirected, such as with rheumatoid arthritis and other illnesses, which can cause swelling, pain, and other symptoms.

In recent years, researchers have learned that inflammation contributes to damage in other parts of the body as well. And diabetes and heart disease are two of these newfound inflammatory conditions. "Diabetes is a chronic inflammatory state," says Judith Stanton, MD, an instructor in the internal medicine residency program at Alameda County Medical Center in California. "Recent research has also linked chronic inflammation to the development of coronary artery disease and heart attack."

Dr. Katz explains that the system recently became more sophisticated with the addition of the concept of glycemic load. "When the glycemic index first came out, some foods high in natural sugars, like carrots, were considered almost as bad as ice cream," he says. "But the glycemic load looks beyond just sugar content to the distribution of sugars within the foods. When you look at foods by their glycemic load, it gives you a better picture of how healthy they are." For more information on utilizing these tools in planning your meals, as well as a database of foods that's searchable by glycemic index and glycemic load, visit glycemicindex.com.

■ **KEEP CHOLESTEROL UNDER CONTROL.** Managing your blood sugar is just one part of the diet equation. The other is getting your cholesterol under control, which means keeping your levels of "bad" LDL cholesterol below 130 and your "good" HDL cholesterol above 40.

Among the hundreds of supposed ways to lower cholesterol, Dr. Katz zeroes in on the following dietary advice: "First, you want to banish the trans fats," he says. "This means looking for the word *hydrogenated* on the labels of processed foods and avoiding them entirely. Also be careful of the saturated fats found in red meat and dairy products, and replace them with the omega-3 fats found in fish and fish oil or the monounsaturated fats from nuts, seeds, and olive oil. And finally, get plenty of fiber from foods like beans, lentils, oats, apples, and berries. Replacing refined grains with high-fiber ones not only helps your blood sugar but your cholesterol as well."

Cholesterol-lowering drugs have also come a long way. "Studies have shown that using cholesterol-lowering medications with type 2 diabetes can reduce by 24 percent the risk of a major cardiovascular event," says Caskey. Ask your doctor if these drugs are right for you.

■ **ENLIST A NUTRITIONIST.** The dietary advice for diabetes and heart disease management may largely overlap, but it's still a massive amount of information to process. That's why Dr. Stanton says one of your best strategies is to see a nutritionist. "If you don't know enough about the proper diabetic diet, make an appointment with a nutritionist because it's the single most important factor in controlling the disease," she says.

The Diabetes Lowdown

Considering obesity's role in both diabetes and heart disease, the pressure to lose weight quickly can be intense. But Judith Stanton, MD, an instructor in the internal medicine residency program at Alameda County Medical Center in California, says that people with diabetes need to be wary of trendy weight-loss strategies. "In the last 2 decades, there was a lot of emphasis on low-fat diets," she says. "This led many people to eat a diet much too high in carbohydrates, which will worsen insulin resistance and the progression of diabetes."

Then the trend shifted toward diet plans that were low in carbohydrates and higher in protein and fat. But Dr. Stanton says that these, too, are not without problems. "High-protein diets put a lot of work on the kidneys, and many diabetics have early kidney disease, although they may not be aware of it," she says. "Extreme high-protein diets can even cause kidney damage or, in some cases, kidney failure."

To avoid these diet pitfalls, Dr. Stanton advises moderation in all things: "Diabetics need to limit but not eliminate carbohydrates and focus on eating complex carbohydrates with a lower glycemic index, in combination with a balanced amount of protein and healthy fats."

■ **PUMP UP YOUR EXERCISE ROUTINE.** With all this focus on food, it's easy to forget the second key component of both diabetes and heart disease management: exercise. Some diabetes patients need to start slowly and work their way safely into a program, so talk to your doctor before beginning a new exercise regimen. "Small changes can add up over time, and the goal is to keep improving," says Caskey. "This might mean starting simple, like parking at the far end of a parking lot to increase your number of steps or meeting a friend once or twice a week to walk together."

■ **STAMP OUT SMOKING.** When you consider that smoking causes more heart-related than lung-related deaths (140,000 compared to 100,000 per year between 1997 and 2001) . . . Do you really need another reason to quit?

High Blood Pressure

FEW HEALTH CONDITIONS are as easy to overlook as high blood pressure. Considering that it causes virtually no symptoms, you may go weeks without giving it a second thought. But when you do stop and think about its effects on the body, it's easy to see why it earns the ominous moniker "the silent killer."

What's the Connection?

While you may not notice any warning signs, high blood pressure, or hypertension, becomes steadily more dangerous as the pressure created when your heart beats (systolic) rises above 120 mm Hg (millimeters of mercury), and the pressure when your heart rests (diastolic) shoots past 80 mm Hg. "When you think about this excess force being applied to all the blood vessels in your body 60 to 80 times a minute, you can begin to understand the trauma that it inflicts," says David L. Katz, MD, MPH, director of the Yale Prevention Research Center in Derby, Connecticut, and author of *The Way to Eat.*

Though it may sound clichéd, trying to figure out what comes first in the relationship between diabetes, blood pressure, and heart disease really is like the old chicken-and-egg debate. People with diabetes are more likely to have high blood pressure, but diabetes can also lead directly to high blood pressure. Same with heart disease: It can be partially caused by the damage done by high blood pressure to the arteries—and by the same token, atherosclerosis can cause blood pressure to rise.

This much is certain: Diabetes packs a one-two punch that puts people with the disease at a much greater risk of developing high blood pressure than the general population. "People with diabetes have obesity, which is also a risk factor for high blood pressure," says Manisha Chandalia, MD, associate professor of internal medicine-endocrinology at the University of Texas Southwestern Medical Center at Dallas. "Diabetes, high blood pressure, and bad lipids are like bad guys who stick together."

What's more, the stress that obesity puts on the blood vessels is made even worse by high levels of sugar floating around in the bloodstream. "Diabetes directly affects blood pressure, as the thicker blood causes more difficulty for the heart to pump the blood," says Daisy Merey, MD, PhD, author of *Don't Be a Slave to What You Crave* and *The Palm Beach Diet Doctor's Prescription*. "Also, there is an elevation of fats in the blood from both obesity and diabetes that destines one to be hypertensive."

Add to this the fact that diabetes often causes kidney disease, while the kidneys play a critical role in lowering blood pressure by filtering impurities out of the blood, and you soon realize how diabetes presents a "perfect storm" to your blood pressure reading (see "The Diabetes Lowdown" on page 59).

How Common Is It?

Considering all that, it's no surprise that people with diabetes have a higher-than-usual risk of developing high blood pressure. But most people are shocked when they learn just how high that risk really is. "Eighteen percent of the general population, or 50 million Americans, have high blood pressure," says Judith Stanton, MD, an instructor in the internal medicine residency program at Alameda County Medical Center in California. "And 73 percent of diabetics have high blood pressure."

Couple that with the fact that 30 to 35 percent of the people who have high blood pressure aren't even aware that they have it, and you get a sense of how high the stakes are.

What Is My Risk?

Having diabetes is one of the greatest risk factors for high blood pressure. But just because diabetes, heart disease, and high blood pressure are intertwined, that isn't all bad. Making a positive change in one area benefits the others, too. "Studies have shown that controlling blood pressure in diabetics can significantly reduce many complications of diabetes, including a 32 percent reduction in death, a 44 percent reduction in stroke, a 56 percent reduction in heart failure, and an almost 40 percent reduction in damage to small vessels that particularly affect the eyes," says Beverly Caskey, RPh, a Medco pharmacist who specializes in diabetes care.

Of course, before you can make a change, you first need to know what risk factors to look for. These questions will help you determine that.

- Is your total cholesterol greater than 200 mg/dL (milligrams per deciliter)?

- Is your BMI (body mass index) greater than 25?

- Is your waistline greater than 34 inches (if you're a woman) or 40 inches (if you're a man)?

- Would you describe yourself as inactive?

- Do you heavily salt your food?

- Have you or your doctor noted decreased kidney function?

- Do you smoke?

- Do you have a family history of high blood pressure?

According to Caskey, "If the answer to any of these questions is yes, then you have a higher risk of high blood pressure." And your risk increases with each yes.

What Should I Watch For?

Like heart disease, one of the most frightening prospects of high blood pressure is that you might not know you have it until damage has already been done. "As with diabetes, the important thing to remember about hypertension is that until it causes a catastrophic event [such as a heart attack or stroke], it has no symptoms, which is why it's often called the silent killer," says Dr. Stanton. "It is therefore extremely important for people to have their blood pressure checked at least once a year to screen for the disease." Our other experts echo that advice.

High blood pressure will on occasion provide you with warning signs that something is awry, including:

⚕ When to See the Doctor

- If you have a home blood pressure reading of greater than 130/85 mm Hg (millimeters of mercury), see your doctor as soon as possible.

- If you have high cholesterol, are overweight, are inactive, smoke, have a family history of high blood pressure, or have decreased kidney function, you need to be under a doctor's supervision for diabetes and blood pressure risk.

- If you have problems with blood pressure and experience headaches, dizziness, flushing, decreased exercise tolerance, shortness of breath, fatigue, or nosebleeds, see your doctor immediately.

- If you have diabetes and high blood pressure, ask your doctor if you should see other specialists, such as a podiatrist or an ophthalmologist.

- Blood pressure reading greater than 130/85 mm Hg
- Headaches
- Dizziness
- Flushed feeling in the face
- Decreased endurance during exercise
- Shortness of breath on exertion
- Fatigue
- Nosebleeds

Because people with diabetes may experience some of these symptoms anyway—particularly fatigue and shortness of breath—they need to be especially diligent about contacting their doctor if blood pressure is a concern.

What Can I Do about It?

It may seem like the odds are stacked against you, but, contrary to the numbers, diabetes and high blood pressure don't have to go hand in hand. And considering the synergistic relationship between heart disease and hypertension, many of the same strategies discussed in Heart Disease (page 44) apply here, too.

Still, some strategies specifically target high blood pressure. These are your weapons in the fight against hypertension.

■ **KNOW YOUR ABCS.** If you already have diabetes, your doctor may already have discussed the ABCs of diabetes care. "These are managing your A1C or blood glucose level, blood pressure, and cholesterol," says Wahida Karmally, RD, director of nutrition at the Irving Center for Clinical Research at Columbia-Presbyterian Medical Center in New York City and a member of the American Heart Association's nutrition committee.

Managing your ABCs is a multifaceted plan that includes diet, exercise, and medication, and positive changes to one component usually carry over to the others as well. "Each one of these is important to reduce, delay, or prevent complications of diabetes, and every single step will help," says Caskey. "Work with your health care team, family, and friends to decide what a reasonable and achievable goal is for you. Concentrate on your successes, and take good care of yourself."

■ **DO THE DASH.** One of the best ways to manage your ABCs is through diet. And though it's a few years old, the DASH (Dietary Approaches to Stop Hypertension) diet remains the gold standard in managing blood pressure through nutrition. Developed by the National Heart, Lung, and Blood Institute (NHLBI), the DASH diet has proven as effective as medication in reducing high blood pressure in several studies. Its basic components are plentiful fruits and vegetables, lots of fiber, low-fat dairy products, and low levels of saturated fat and cholesterol. Here's a quick overview of the roughly 2,000-calorie-a-day plan.

RESEARCH BUZZ

Balancing BP Drugs and Glucose Control

Medication is a critical part of many blood pressure–reducing strategies. But recent research suggests that some beta-blockers, a common blood pressure–lowering medication, may actually increase levels of blood glucose in people with diabetes.

To test this theory, researchers evaluated 1,235 people between the ages of 36 and 85 with type 2 diabetes. The participants were divided into two groups and each given a different beta-blocker: Half took carvedilol, and half took metoprolol. At the end of nearly 4 years, the researchers discovered that both beta-blockers were well tolerated, but people who took carvedilol had lower blood sugar levels than those who took metoprolol.

Though more long-term study is needed, you may want to ask your doctor if carvedilol is preferable to metoprolol if you have diabetes and high blood pressure. In addition, two other blood pressure medications commonly prescribed to people with diabetes, angiotensin II receptor blockers (ARBs) and ACE (angiotensin-converting enzyme) inhibitors, do not appear to adversely affect blood sugar and even help protect kidney function.

- Grains, including whole grain bread, rice, pasta, or cereal: 7 or 8 servings

- Vegetables, particularly raw and leafy choices: 4 or 5 servings

- Low-fat dairy products, including milk and yogurt: 2 or 3 servings

- Lean meats, such as poultry and fish: 2 or fewer servings

In addition, these tips will help you meet the diet's goals.

- Eat one or two vegetarian meals a week.

- Trim your portions of meat by one-third or one-half.

- Add an extra serving of fruits and vegetables at lunch and dinner to get more of these foods.

- Snack on raw vegetables, plain popcorn, yogurt, raisins, and nuts.

- Cut butter and margarine consumption by half.

RUN THE NUMBERS OFTEN. The asymptomatic nature of high blood pressure means that the only way to know where you stand is to get it checked. Luckily, this is easier than ever, and you don't have to go to a doctor's office to do it. "I recommend checking your blood pressure at home from time to time," says Dr. Chandalia. "If it is ever more than 130/85, contact your doctor."

TAKE YOUR MEDICATION. Amid all the focus on prevention, it's easy to overlook just how greatly medication can help manage blood pressure. "Medications often will help in surprising ways, such as those that reduce blood pressure and also protect the kidneys," says Caskey. "Drugs in this category are called angiotensin-converting enzyme [ACE] inhibitors and angiotensin II receptor blockers [ARBs]."

STAMP OUT THE SALT. Though the message has been mixed over the years, the DASH diet studies by the NHLBI, among others, reveal a clear connection between high sodium intake and high blood pressure. The recommended daily value of sodium is 2,400 milligrams, or a little less than a

The Diabetes Lowdown

Diabetes. Obesity. Heart disease. High blood pressure. If diabetes research has taught us anything, it's that these four factors are almost always intertwined. Recent research indicates that we may need to add another to that list: kidney disease.

When you have diabetes, the stress on the small blood vessels can prevent your kidneys from cleaning your blood properly. In addition, bladder problems can cause urine to back up and injure your kidneys, eventually leading to kidney disease. And because your kidneys are no longer properly filtering your blood, these extra impurities contribute to high blood pressure, completing the cycle.

If you have diabetes and high blood pressure, make sure to ask your doctor about your kidney function. With regular screenings, kidney problems can be easily detected and prevented.

---

teaspoon, but most people consume around 4,000 milligrams. And the DASH diet showed the best blood pressure–lowering results at a minuscule 1,500 milligrams of sodium.

The NHLBI has dozens of great tips for reducing salt intake at their Web site: nhlbi.nih.gov/hbp/prevent/sodium/sodium.htm. Just a handful of these include using fresh foods whenever possible, choosing low-salt options for canned or processed foods, rinsing canned foods with water to remove some of the salt, and flavoring dishes with herbs instead of salt.

■ **KEEP AN "EYE" ON OTHER BODY PARTS.** The heart isn't the only body part at risk for damage from high blood pressure. The kidneys, feet, and eyes are among others that also rely on good circulation. "Diabetics need to take great care not to injure themselves, especially in the lower extremities," says Fred Pescatore, MD, a traditionally trained physician practicing nutritional medicine and the author of *The Hamptons Diet*. "They should also see a foot doctor regularly to ensure proper foot care, as well as see an ophthalmologist on a regular basis. High blood pressure in the diabetic could lead to earlier risks for glaucoma and bleeding in the retina, which can lead to blindness."

■ **FIT IN FITNESS.** Not surprisingly, exercise is key for controlling high blood pressure, just as it is for managing diabetes. And if it's been years since you've exercised, even small, gradual changes in your routine can help. "Take the stairs instead of the elevator. Stretch for 10 minutes when you wake up in the morning. Do small tasks and chores during commercials. Find an activity that you enjoy that makes your body move," says Caskey. "Consistent change over time will make a difference. Before starting an exercise program, check with your doctor first to make sure you can start safely."

■ **TRY THE RIGHT SUPPLEMENTS.** Dr. Pescatore says that a handful of nutritional supplements—under your doctor's supervision—can also play a role in blood pressure management. These include magnesium orotate or magnesium taurate (500 to 1,000 milligrams three times a day); taurine, which acts as a natural diuretic (1,000 milligrams three times a day); and fish oil (1,000 to 2,000 milligrams a day in divided doses).

Kidney Disease

HAVING DIABETES MEANS the choices you make today have direct consequences on your quality of life later, sometimes in ways you might not immediately associate with blood sugar. Consider your kidneys, for example: The food you eat, whether or not you exercise, the medications you take, if you smoke, and how well you manage your blood sugar and blood pressure—all the aspects of diabetes care—make a major impact on these two bean-shaped organs.

What's the Connection?

Diabetes is the leading cause of kidney failure in the United States and in developing countries around the world, accounting for 50 percent of all cases, says Thomas Hostetter, MD, professor of nephrology at Albert Einstein College of Medicine in the Bronx and chair of the American Society of Nephrology's Kidney Disease Advisory Group.

Your kidneys perform a vital life process. They filter wastes and extra water from about 200 quarts of blood a day, turning it into urine and sending it to your bladder so it can leave your body. While they filter out the things your body doesn't need, they retain what's necessary (such as sodium, potassium, and phosphorus) before sending your blood back into circulation.

Diabetes can interfere with this process. Higher-than-normal blood glucose levels damage the endothelial cells that line the blood vessels in your kidneys and throughout your body. This situation also creates oxidative stress, in which free radicals damage cells, which can lead to disease, says Robert C. Stanton, MD, principal investigator in the section on vascular cell biology and the chief of the nephrology section at Joslin Clinic at the Joslin Diabetes Center in Boston and associate professor of medicine at Harvard Medical School. Diabetes also increases the filtration rate in the kidneys, which heightens the pressure inside the blood vessels that nourish the kidneys' filters.

In addition, people with diabetes have higher levels of an enzyme called protein kinase C beta. "It's one of a number of mechanisms that we know are involved in all diabetes complications, including kidney disease," Dr. Stanton says. Another enzyme, transforming growth factor beta, has been shown animal studies to be an important factor in kidney scarring. Elevated levels of sugar-coated proteins called advance glycation end products also cause cellular damage in the kidneys. Each of these factors can lead to kidney disease, Dr. Stanton explains.

When your kidneys become damaged, they're less able to manage their many tasks. These workhorse organs help regulate levels of body fluid; sodium, potassium, and acid-base; red blood cells; and the hormones responsible for maintaining healthy bones. When kidney function falls below 10 to 15 percent, you need dialysis—a method of removing toxins from the blood—or a kidney transplant.

Making matters worse, millions of people don't know they have diabetes and are walking around with chronically high blood sugar and unknowingly damaging their kidneys. Of the 20.8 million people with diabetes, experts estimate that only about 14.6 million are diagnosed, leaving more than 6 million undiagnosed.

How Common Is It?

As diabetes becomes more common, so does kidney disease, or diabetic nephropathy. The number of people with kidney disease is doubling every decade, according to the American Society of Nephrology. Today, a person with type 1 or type 2 diabetes has a 30 to 40 percent chance of developing some level of kidney disease, Dr. Stanton says. "There's been a massive increase in kidney disease in the last 20 years, driven mostly by diabetes," he says.

It's been assumed that people with type 1 diabetes are at high risk for kidney disease, and experts believed people who had type 2 had a lower risk. But that's likely because people with type 2 were dying earlier from heart disease, Dr. Stanton says. Now that medicine is helping people live longer with heart disease and high blood pressure, type 2 diabetes patients are getting kidney disease.

What Is My Risk?

To get an idea of your kidneys' future health, consider these questions.

1. Do you test your blood sugar at home every day?

2. Is your blood sugar under control with diet and/or medications?

3. Is your blood pressure less than 130/80 mm Hg (millimeters of mercury)?

4. Is your BMI (body mass index) in a healthy range of 18.5 to 25?

5. Are your cholesterol levels within target ranges? (Total cholesterol should be below 200 mg/dL; for more information, see page 68.)

6. Are you a nonsmoker?

■ **YOU ANSWERED NO TO QUESTION 1:** Now-and-then testing puts your kidneys at risk. If you don't test regularly, you won't know if high blood sugar levels are damaging your kidneys.

■ **YOU ANSWERED YES TO ALL SIX QUESTIONS:** You're doing a good job of protecting your kidneys from damage. Keeping your blood sugar levels within a healthy range is crucial for preventing kidney disease, as are healthy blood pressure, BMI, and cholesterol numbers. And avoiding cigarettes means you're not exposing your blood vessels to more damage.

■ **YOU ANSWERED YES TO MORE THAN THREE QUESTIONS:** You're on your way to providing your kidneys with optimum protection. You probably know the areas you should be working on, whether it's doing a better job of monitoring your blood sugar, reducing your blood pressure, or losing weight. It's worth the effort to keep your kidneys healthy.

■ **YOU ANSWERED NO TO MORE THAN THREE QUESTIONS:** You probably didn't need to take this quiz to learn that you must make some changes in your life. Reach out to your doctor, a nutritionist, or a diabetes educator for help in turning all those nos to kidney-friendly yeses.

What Should I Watch For?

Diabetes-related kidney damage happens very slowly and may not be evident until the kidneys lose almost all of their function. At that point, symptoms finally surface: fatigue, nausea, and swollen hands and feet. To avoid that situation, see your doctor for regular testing—it's the only way to confirm that your kidneys are in good shape. The following tests help your doctor monitor your kidney function.

■ **CREATININE AND GFR:** Once a year, get your blood tested for creatinine, a waste product of muscle that's a good marker of kidney function. It builds up in your blood if your kidneys aren't functioning properly. Dr. Stanton urges you to go one step further: Ask your doctor to check your glomerular filtration rate, which reveals how fast your creatinine levels are changing over time. The GFR more accurately reflects your kidney function than does the serum creatinine level alone, he says.

■ **MICROALBUMINURIA TEST:** This screens for a small increase of the protein albumin in a urine sample and should be done at least once a year, Dr. Stanton says. Studies show that as albumin levels rise, so does the risk for cardiovascular disease and kidney disease, whether or not you have diabetes. But many people miss this important information: Surveys show that only 60 to 70 percent of people with diabetes get the test regularly, says Dr. Hostetter.

■ **HEMOGLOBIN A1C:** This blood test tells your doctor how well you're controlling your blood sugar over time by averaging your blood glucose for 2 to 3 months. Doctors recommend having this done two to four times a year.

When to See the Doctor

If you've been diagnosed with diabetes, your doctor will begin testing and monitoring the health of your kidneys. You don't need to see a kidney specialist at this point, says Thomas Hostetter, MD, professor of nephrology at Albert Einstein College of Medicine in the Bronx and chair of the American Society of Nephrology's Kidney Disease Advisory Group. However, if your glomerular filtration rate falls to 30, which means you have 30 percent of your kidney function, you should see a kidney specialist, he says.

What Can I Do about It?

■ **MONITOR YOUR BLOOD SUGAR.** There's no way to control your blood sugar levels unless you test your blood every day, starting as soon as you're diagnosed and even if you're not taking medication, says Stanley Mirsky, MD, an endocrinologist at Lenox Hill Hospital in New York City and co-author of *Diabetes Survival Guide*. You'll need a blood glucose monitor, test strips, and a small lancet to prick your finger. These supplies are available at your doctor's office or a pharmacy.

If you keep your blood sugar within normal levels with diet alone, check your blood once before breakfast, he says. If you're taking hypoglycemic drugs, add a test before dinner. If you take insulin, include a bedtime check (that's a total of three tests). And anytime your levels are too high, you're ill, or you feel very thirsty and are urinating more often, check your blood *four* times a day: before breakfast, lunch, and dinner and at bedtime.

It's also essential to keep a record of your results. This will show you how your body responds to what you're eating and guide you in tweaking your diet, Dr. Mirsky says. Share the log with your physician, who may use it to adjust your medication or make suggestions for changes to your diet or activity level. Keeping an eye on your blood sugar levels helps you stay on track. "People need to be reminded that they have diabetes, and checking their sugar levels reminds them," Dr. Mirsky says.

■ **STRIVE FOR PERFECTION.** "If you control your blood sugar perfectly, all evidence says that it will help prevent kidney damage," Dr. Hostetter says. When Canadian researchers used an A1C test to measure the long-term blood sugar control of 100 people with diabetes on kidney dialysis, they found that most of those patients had poor glycemic control and also suffered heart and blood vessel problems.

Every time you lower your A1C test results by 1 percentage point (say, from 8 percent to 7 percent), you lower your risk of microvascular complications, including kidney disease, by 40 percent, according to the Centers for Disease Control and Prevention. (Microvascular complications are those that involve the tiny blood vessels in your body.) Dr Mirsky offers four simple rules for blood sugar control.

- Stick with one starch per meal. If you're having a potato with dinner, don't have a piece of bread. Is corn on your plate? Skip the rice.

- Only eat soup you can see through. Opaque soups such as broccoli Cheddar, potato, pea, and lentil have added flour and starches that add up to a carb overload. Choose chicken noodle or vegetable soup instead.

- Skip apples and pineapples. They have too many carbs for one sitting, Dr. Mirsky says. The exception: It's okay to eat apples if you're an avid exerciser, you take insulin, or your diabetes is mild.

- Limit fruits to two servings a day. But if you're taking insulin, it's okay to have another for an afternoon snack.

■ **GET A HANDLE ON HIGH BLOOD PRESSURE.** Diabetes is the number one cause of kidney disease, but hypertension ranks as number two. Having high blood pressure damages the waste-filtering blood vessels in your kidneys. "High blood pressure may be more damaging to people with diabetes than people without diabetes," Dr. Hostetter says.

Controlling your blood pressure lowers your risk of microvascular complications such as kidney and nerve disease by about 33 percent, according to the CDC. Every 10 mm Hg drop in your systolic blood pressure (the top number) lowers your risk for diabetes complications by 12 percent. When you have diabetes, aim for a blood pressure of 130/80 mm Hg or lower. Your blood pressure should be taken at every doctor's visit or at least once a year.

■ **ASK ABOUT ACE INHIBITORS AND ARBS.** Doctors can now prescribe a blood pressure medication that helps your kidneys. Angiotensin-converting enzyme (ACE) inhibitors and angiotensin II receptor blockers (ARBs) help lower your blood pressure and protect your kidneys more than other drugs do. "It's the main way we can slow the progression of kidney disease," Dr. Hostetter says.

Everyone with diabetes and high blood pressure should take an ACE inhibitor or an ARB. Research suggests these drugs are also worth taking for kidney damage alone, Dr. Hostetter says. (Most people with kidney damage do have high blood pressure, however.) Researchers are looking at whether or not combining an ACE inhibitor and an ARB for treatment will be beneficial.

■ **DROP EXTRA POUNDS.** Being obese triples your risk of chronic kidney failure, according to the American Society of Nephrology. But if you lose just 10 percent of your body weight, you can significantly improve your blood sugar levels, which will help you avoid kidney disease.

A study in New Zealand tested the effects of different diets on 93 women who were overweight and resistant to insulin. They were split into three groups that each ate a different diet for a year: high-protein, high-carb/high-fiber, or high-fat. Not surprisingly, the women on the high-protein and high-carb/high-fiber diets dropped pounds, particularly around their waists, and were better able to handle glucose. The women on the high-fat diet gained weight around their middles. To emulate the trimmer women, fill your plate with high-fiber vegetables and fruit, lean meat, low-fat dairy products, and whole grains.

■ **BRING DOWN HIGH CHOLESTEROL.** Research has found that people with high cholesterol are more likely to lose kidney function. The Joslin Diabetes Center recommends getting your cholesterol checked once a year and aiming for a "bad" LDL cholesterol level of 70 mg/dL (milligrams per deciliter) if you have diabetes or heart disease. Aim for a "good" HDL level of higher than 40 mg/dL (for men) or 50 mg/dL (for women). Total cholesterol should be less than 200 mg/dL, and triglyceride levels should be less than 150 mg/dL. Eating foods low in saturated and trans fats will help you meet those goals. That means less red meat, whole-milk dairy products, deep-fried foods, and anything processed or packaged (such as baked goods and snack foods).

■ **CONSIDER CUTTING BACK ON PROTEIN.** Some doctors recommend that people with diabetes restrict protein because damaged kidneys may not properly separate protein from wastes in the blood, but this is a controversial subject. "Many people say it hasn't been studied as well as it should be," Dr. Hostetter says.

And protein restriction is not easy. Protein is not only in meat but also in other foods, including vegetables. And restricting protein too much can be dangerous, Dr. Hostetter says. If you decide you want to limit your protein, get help from a nutritionist or diabetes educator. "We don't think people should try it on their own," he says.

■ **COMMIT TO QUIT IF YOU SMOKE.** High blood glucose already wreaks havoc on the endothelial cells that line the blood vessels in your kidneys. When you smoke cigarettes, you're poisoning cells even more, Dr. Stanton says.

How can you quit? Experts suggest finding something else to do what cigarettes normally do for you. If you smoke to relax, take up yoga and learn deep breathing. If smoking revs you up, take a walk or start exercising for energy. You can try to quit cold turkey, but your doctor can also talk to you about over-the-counter and prescription drugs that can help you on your way to a smoke-free life.

Liver Disease

A DIAGNOSIS OF TYPE 2 DIABETES usually comes with the message that controlling your disease will help you avoid well-known related complications. Your doctor most likely briefed you on heart disease, neuropathy, and eye disease, so those issues may be at the forefront of your mind. But have you given any thought lately to your liver?

Your liver is the largest organ in your body and plays an essential role in your health. It removes poisons from your blood, helps control infections, regulates blood clotting, and makes bile, which absorbs fats and fat-soluble vitamins. But if your liver becomes infected or inflamed from a virus, bacteria, or chemical changes in your body, it can't do its job well. That can lead to cirrhosis, a condition in which healthy liver tissue turns to scar tissue and blocks blood flow, preventing your liver from working properly.

Many people associate liver disease with alcoholics because years of alcohol abuse damage this vital organ. But diabetes is also a major contributor to liver disease—not because of too much alcohol but from a buildup of fat in the liver. The result is called nonalcoholic fatty liver disease, the most common chronic liver disease in the United States—and it's most prevalent among people with diabetes.

What's the Connection?

Doctors aren't sure exactly why people with diabetes are at higher risk for liver disease or how the liver becomes fatty. You don't just eat hamburgers and end up with a fatty liver. Overeating does play a role, but so does insulin resistance, says Gerald Bernstein, MD, director of the Gerald J. Friedman Diabetes Institute Diabetes Management Program at Beth Israel Hospital in New York City. Being less sensitive to insulin means your body has chronically high blood sugar, which wreaks havoc on many of your organs and body systems, including your liver.

Fatty liver is practically unavoidable if you have diabetes. "If you were to do ultrasounds on people with diabetes, you would find increased fat in the liver, even in people who have fairly controlled diabetes," Dr. Bernstein says. Impaired glucose tolerance, or prediabetes, sets the process in motion years—even a decade—before you're diagnosed with diabetes. When fat stays in the liver for a very long time, you develop liver disease.

Studies have found that some people with type 2 diabetes have abnormally high levels of liver enzymes. Enzymes usually remain in the liver, but when they leak into the blood, it's a sign that the organ is damaged. Four clinical trials found that as many as 24 percent of the 3,701 diabetic people screened had more than the normal amount of liver enzymes.

Doctors continue to study which comes first: liver disease or diabetes, says Jeanne M. Clark, MD, associate professor of medicine and epidemiology at Johns Hopkins University in Baltimore. Some studies show that people with fatty liver disease are more likely to develop diabetes. But research also shows that if you already have diabetes, you're still at higher risk of developing liver disease and cirrhosis than the general population, even if you currently have a healthy liver, she says.

Factors that put you at risk for getting type 2 diabetes—including being overweight or obese, having high blood pressure, and having high cholesterol—also put you at risk for liver disease. "And if you're overweight and have hepatitis C, a major cause of liver disease and cirrhosis, you're more likely to get cirrhosis," Dr. Clark says. The virus causes inflammation and long-term, low-grade damage to the liver.

How Common Is It?

Diabetes is the single most common cause of liver disease in the United States, and cirrhosis is the fourth-leading cause of death among people with diabetes. Studies show that 34 to 74 percent of people with diabetes have nonalcoholic fatty liver disease. Among people who are obese and have diabetes, the prevalence of nonalcoholic fatty liver disease nears 100 percent.

Doctors have also found that people with diabetes are more likely to carry the hepatitis C virus than people who don't have diabetes. About 4 percent of people with diabetes have hepatitis C antibodies, compared with only 1.6 percent of the general population. Doctors think hepatitis C may lead to diabetes because the virus seems to impair insulin receptors.

What Is My Risk?

To assess your risk, consider these questions.

1. Does your blood sugar regularly go out of the normal, healthy range?

2. Are you overweight or obese?

3. Is your waist circumference more than 35 inches (if you're a woman) or 40 inches (if you're a man)?

4. Do you have high cholesterol (240 mg/dL or above)?

■ **YOU ANSWERED NO TO ALL FOUR QUESTIONS:** You're doing a good job at protecting your liver from disease and cirrhosis.

■ **YOU ANSWERED NO TO TWO OR THREE QUESTIONS:** You're doing all right, but you still need to work on protecting your liver. Losing weight (particularly around your middle), doing a better job of controlling your blood sugar, and keeping your cholesterol in a healthy range will actually reduce the amount of fat that accumulates in your liver.

■ **YOU ANSWERED YES TO THREE OR FOUR QUESTIONS:** There's no way around it—if you want to protect your liver, you have to work harder to get your blood sugar under control, lower your cholesterol, and lose weight and abdominal fat.

What Should I Watch For?

There aren't any symptoms in the early stage of liver disease other than a vague feeling of fatigue and not feeling well, Dr. Clark says. If the disease progresses to cirrhosis, you'll notice more fluid retention in your abdomen or legs, she says.

What Can I Do about It?

■ **CONTINUE TO MONITOR AND CONTROL YOUR BLOOD SUGAR.** As with so many other diabetes complications, one of the best things you can do to protect yourself against liver disease is to control your blood sugar. "Elevated

---

⚕ When to See the Doctor

If you experience fatigue, malaise, and a dull ache in your upper right abdomen, see your doctor—they're all associated with nonalcoholic fatty liver disease.

It's unlikely you'll have symptoms in the early stages of liver disease, however. If you have diabetes, your doctor probably tests for liver enzymes as part of the metabolic panel when you have blood work, says Jeanne M. Clark, MD, associate professor of medicine and epidemiology at Johns Hopkins University in Baltimore. And if you're taking cholesterol medication, which can increase liver enzymes in your blood, your doctor will automatically monitor your liver function.

blood sugar is like a poison," Dr. Bernstein says. In one study of 175 people with type 1 or type 2 diabetes in Finland, 57 percent of those who had an abnormal liver functioning test were more likely to be obese and have poor control of their blood sugar.

■ **AS ALWAYS, AIM FOR A HEALTHY WEIGHT.** Losing 5 to 10 percent of your overall weight can substantially lower your risk of liver disease and other diabetes complications, Dr. Clark says. Eating healthy foods and getting exercise every day can lower inflammation in your liver, reduce the amount of liver enzymes in your blood, and make your body more sensitive to insulin.

More than 70 percent of people with nonalcoholic fatty liver disease are obese, according to the Mayo Clinic, and experts say your risk increases with every extra pound you carry around. If you have a body mass index of more than 25, diet and exercise can actually lower the amount of fat that's accumulated in your liver. Some good rules to follow: Eat high-fiber foods such as fruits, vegetables, and whole grains and only a small amount of saturated fat. Your total fat intake shouldn't make up more than 30 percent of your total calories.

■ **WHITTLE YOUR WAIST.** Having fat around your middle puts you at higher risk of liver disease, Dr. Clark says. Researchers measuring abdominal fat found that having a waist circumference of more than 62 inches makes a person more likely to have nonalcoholic fatty liver disease. A healthy waist circumference is 40 inches or less for a man and 35 inches or less for a woman, Dr. Clark says.

Working up a little sweat may offer the best way to slim down your midsection. Compared with dieting, exercise seems to have more of an effect on abdominal fat, Dr. Clark says, and it doesn't have to be very intense for you to reap benefits. Moderate exercise such as brisk walking has been shown to help reduce belly fat.

■ **EAT LIKE YOU'RE IN THE MEDITERRANEAN.** A healthy diet should always be part of your diabetes-control plan, and some observational studies suggest that a Mediterranean diet in particular may help protect against liver disease, Dr. Clark says. The emphasis on monounsaturated fats and low-glycemic carbohydrates is healthier for your liver. Use olive oil as your main fat source (steer clear of saturated and trans fats), and fill up on foods like fruits, vegetables, bread, cereal, potatoes, beans, nuts, seeds, fish, poultry, and low-fat dairy products. Mediterranean diets include very little red meat and limit eggs to four a week.

■ **DEVELOP A DOABLE DIET.** Adjusting your eating habits in ways you can sustain for years is more important than getting hung up on a particular diet, Dr. Clark says. You need a long-term plan to maintain a healthy weight and lower your risk for diabetes complications. And very restrictive diets definitely won't do your liver any good. Studies have found that rapid weight loss may lead to inflammation of the liver, death of liver cells, and fibrosis, in which scar tissue forms because of infection or inflammation.

You'll get bigger health benefits by making small changes. Ease into healthier eating by switching to fat-free milk from whole, eating more grilled chicken and fish and less red meat, adding more side dishes, preparing healthy meals at home rather than eating out, and leaving a few bites of food on your plate rather than leaving it squeaky clean.

■ **CURB HIGH CHOLESTEROL.** Up to 80 percent of people with nonalcoholic fatty liver disease have high cholesterol—but lower it to a healthy level, and you can stabilize or even reverse liver disease. Exercising, eating less saturated and trans fats and more monounsaturated sources (think Mediterranean again), not smoking, and maintaining a healthy weight will help you gain control of your cholesterol, according to the American Diabetes Association.

■ **DON'T TIPPLE IF YOU'RE NOT IN TIP-TOP SHAPE.** Although people with diabetes don't tend to have alcohol-related liver disease, that doesn't mean you can drink cosmopolitans or beer all night. "The more insults you throw at the liver, the worse off you are," Dr. Clark says. It's a double whammy if you have nonalcoholic fatty liver disease and drink alcohol on top of it, she says.

If you're obese, you should watch your alcohol intake even more, because people who are obese and drink at moderate or heavy levels are more at risk for alcohol liver disease, notes Dr. Clark. And, of course, drinking too much alcohol isn't very good for your blood sugar levels, either.

The bottom line: Drink alcohol only if you haven't been diagnosed with nonalcoholic fatty liver disease; your blood sugars are under control; and you don't have other problems that could be affected by alcohol, such as nerve damage. Never drink on an empty stomach—it can cause low blood sugar. Instead, indulge only with meals, and stick to one drink a day if you're a woman, two if you're a man.

■ **DON'T OD ON OTCS.** Following the label instructions on aspirin, ibuprofen, and acetaminophen is safe, even if you have mild liver disease. But overdosing, which isn't hard to do, can be toxic to your liver. A study by researchers at the University of Washington found that overdosing on a pain reliever is the most common cause of sudden liver failure in the United States. Women in particular seem to be vulnerable because they take acetaminophen more often, and their bodies may break down the drug's toxic by-product more slowly, exposing their livers to the harmful substances longer.

Be sure not to exceed the recommended daily dosage, and wait the proper amount of time between doses. Also, be aware that acetaminophen is found in more than 100 over-the-counter medications, including cold and flu remedies, insomnia drugs, allergy medications, and more. Never use one of those along with Tylenol or another acetaminophen-containing drug. If you have cirrhosis, it's important to adjust your dose—or don't take the medications at all, Dr. Clark says.

Urinary Incontinence

THERE'S A SECRET women need to stop keeping.

It's about leaking urine when you sneeze or laugh, having a sudden urge to go but not making it to the bathroom in time, or suddenly urinating without any warning at all.

It's easy to think you're the only one, but urinary incontinence happens to literally millions of people—an estimated 13 million Americans. A large majority—more than 11 million—are women. Almost half of all middle-aged or older women leak urine, yet no one talks about it; many women are too embarrassed to even seek help. In fact, 43 percent of women with the problem put off consulting a doctor for nearly 7 years, according to the National Association for Continence. The real shame is that they're suffering needlessly for years—sometimes decades. Urinary incontinence is very easy to treat.

Some may think losing bladder control simply comes with being a woman. It's true that pregnancy, childbirth, and low estrogen levels at menopause—which can dry out the tissues of the urethra and make the sphincter muscles surrounding the urethra weaker and less likely to close—can contribute to incontinence. But there's another major risk factor that can affect both women and men: diabetes. Research has even shown that incontinence is more prevalent in people with prediabetes. It's time to break the silence and get the help you need.

What's the Connection?

Incontinence is significantly more common among women who have diabetes than among those who don't, and it tends to occur earlier and with more severity. But men with diabetes are also at high risk—maybe even higher than women. One study in Turkey found that 74 percent of the men with diabetes had some degree of bladder dysfunction.

Doctors don't yet fully understand why people who have diabetes are more likely to deal with incontinence, but one theory is that the increased amount of urine from high blood sugar levels may contribute to the problem. Diabetes also increases the risk of urinary tract infections, which can cause incontinence, says Elizabeth Kavaler, MD, a urologist at New York Urological Associates and author of *A Seat on the Aisle, Please!*

If high blood sugar levels have damaged your nerves, you may develop overflow incontinence, which means you're less sensitive to the sensation of a full bladder, Dr. Kavaler says. Your bladder then fills to the point that it literally overflows. It also stretches to hold much more than it should and urine drips out, she says.

If you're a woman with diabetes, you're also more prone to two other types of incontinence: urge and stress incontinence. The first type refers to a sudden urge to go *right now*, then dribbling on the way to the bathroom. Running water or cold temperatures may trigger it. If you have an overactive bladder, you'll feel the urge more often than normal, including in the middle of the night, even if there's not much urine in your bladder. If you have stress incontinence, you tend to leak whenever your bladder feels pressure, such as when you sneeze, laugh, cough, or exercise. Both types apply in your case? That's called mixed incontinence.

Diabetes and incontinence also share a risk factor—obesity, says Larrian Gillespie, MD, a urologist and urogynecologist in Beverly Hills, California, and author of *You Don't Have to Live with Cystitis*. Extra weight puts more pressure on your bladder so that you leak more easily. Taking diuretics or water pills for high blood pressure can also pose problems. These drugs pull water out of the body and dump it in the bladder in high volumes, Dr. Kavaler says, creating a sudden urge to urinate that leads to leaking.

How Common Is It?

When Norwegian researchers surveyed more than 20,000 women, they found urge and mixed incontinence occurred in 39 percent of the women with diabetes, compared with 26 percent of women without diabetes—a 50 percent increased risk. Other studies suggest that urinary incontinence may be up to twice as prevalent in women who have diabetes.

You don't need full-blown diabetes to suffer these consequences. After analyzing 1,461 women for one study, the researchers found that women with prediabetes, as well as diabetes, were significantly more likely to have urge and/or stress incontinence at least once a week, compared with women with normal fasting glucose levels. These women were also more likely to say that incontinence significantly affected their daily activities.

There isn't as much data about men with incontinence as there is for women, but a 2006 study in the *Journal of Urology* found that 17 percent of American men overall experience incontinence (whether or not they have diabetes). The prevalence increased as the men got older, from 11 percent among men ages 60 to 64 to 31 percent for age 85 and older.

What Is My Risk?

With half of all middle-aged and older women experiencing urinary incontinence, it's admittedly not easy to avoid if you're a woman. But your answers to these questions can help you figure out which half you'll likely fall into.

1. Do you have diabetes or prediabetes?

2. Are you obese?

3. Did your mother have incontinence?

IF YOU ANSWERED YES TO ALL THREE: You may be at higher risk for incontinence because of the diabetes/obesity combination as well as a genetic component: If your mother had incontinence, you might, too.

IF YOU ANSWERED YES TO LESS THAN THREE: You may be at lower risk thanks to fewer of the major factors. Still, other issues contribute to incontinence, including pregnancy and childbirth, so it's hard to predict if you'll avoid it.

What Should I Watch For?

There's really no mistaking actual incontinence, but other bladder issues can alert you to an impending problem. People who have diabetes are prone to chronic bladder infections from holding in urine for too long, which can lead to incontinence, Dr. Gillespie says. And if you haven't been diagnosed with diabetes, chronic bladder infections may be a sign of high blood sugar levels. Dr. Gillespie has had patients who didn't know they had diabetes until recurrent bladder infections prompted her to get them tested.

What Can I Do about It?

MAINTAIN HEALTHY BLOOD SUGAR LEVELS. Keep your blood sugar under control, and you can avoid nerve damage that may lead to overflow

---

⚕ When to See the Doctor

If you've begun leaking urine, take notes on how often and when it happens. This will help your doctor determine the kind of incontinence you're experiencing.

Your doctor might also test your urine for a bladder infection and give you a pelvic exam to look for pelvic organ prolapse, a condition in which the pelvic organs hang down into the vaginal canal, causing stress incontinence. Other tests—such as blood tests, pelvic ultrasound, and x-rays—can help determine what kind of incontinence you have.

incontinence. You know the routine: Take your medications, eat a diabetes-friendly diet, and get regular exercise.

■ **EASE THE WEIGHT ON YOUR BLADDER.** You're well aware that if you're at a healthy weight, you'll better manage your blood sugar levels—and maybe even avoid diabetes if you don't yet have it. But here's another reason to drop excess pounds: If you're obese, you're four times more likely to be incontinent than a normal-weight woman is—but lose the weight and you'll improve incontinence.

One study found that a 5 to 10 percent weight loss reduced urinary incontinence just as well as nonsurgical treatments did. Researchers at the University of California, San Francisco, studied 40 overweight or obese women who leaked urine at least four times a week. Half began a weight loss plan immediately, and half held off for 3 months. After losing 35 pounds, the early dieters saw a 60 percent improvement in incontinence, compared with just 15 percent for the late starters. But after the second group began shedding pounds, their symptoms improved 71 percent. The benefits lasted for the 6 months that the researchers continued to track the women.

■ **SCHEDULE PREVENTIVE BATHROOM TRIPS.** If overflow incontinence is your problem, Dr. Gillespie suggests using the bathroom every 3 hours, whether you think you need to or not. Because nerve damage prevents you from feeling the urge to go, you'll have to watch the clock to ensure your bladder doesn't spill over.

■ **STAVE OFF BLADDER INFECTIONS.** An over-the-counter natural remedy called Cystex can help prevent bladder infections, which can cause urgency, says Dr. Gillespie. If you have chronic bladder infections, she recommends taking it every day.

■ **MAKE TIME FOR KEGELS.** Contracting your pelvic muscles with Kegel exercises will help strengthen them and give you more bladder control if you have urge or stress incontinence. To get into the habit of doing them every day, designate a certain time for them, such as while driving to and from work or when you shower. It takes less than 5 minutes three times a day, and doctors say you should notice better bladder control in 3 to 6 weeks.

Here's how to do this simple move: Relax your stomach and legs, then contract the same muscles you'd use to stop the flow of urine while using the bathroom and to stop passing gas. Squeeze these pelvic-floor muscles for three counts, then relax for three counts, without holding your breath. That's one Kegel. Work up to doing 10 to 15 at a time in three separate daily sessions.

■ **SUPPRESS THE URGE.** If you have urge incontinence, try a technique called urge suppression. Instead of immediately fleeing to the bathroom, stay put and quickly tighten and relax your pelvic-floor muscles—the same ones you use for Kegels—several times. At the same time, take deep breaths and try to distract yourself, such as mentally going over your grocery or Christmas shopping list until the urge passes.

You may also want to time bathroom trips for every 1 to $1\frac{1}{2}$ hours. In between, suppress any urges and ignore any leaks while you train your body to wait until the appointed time. As you improve, increase the time between bathroom trips by half an hour.

■ **CONSIDER BIOFEEDBACK THERAPY.** If Kegels and urge suppression aren't helping, talk to your doctor about biofeedback therapy. It works by hooking up sensors to your stomach and inserting a small probe into your vagina.

When you tighten your pelvic muscles, a machine measures the intensity, which shows up as colored lines on a screen. This can help you learn to use the right muscles, and it's so effective that Medicare covers it. There's also a version of this therapy for men.

■ **LET THIRST DICTATE FLUID INTAKE.** "There's a huge water consumption frenzy, telling people to drink and drink and drink," Dr. Kavaler says. As a result, some women simply drink too much and become incontinent. Other women drink inconsistently, drinking little all day and then, say, downing a few liters of water after work, she notes. This fluid version of feast or famine will only irritate your bladder. A better choice: Simply drink whenever you're thirsty throughout the day.

■ **STOP DRINKING 3 HOURS BEFORE BEDTIME.** If you go to bed at 10 PM, don't drink after 7 to avoid nighttime episodes, Dr. Gillespie says.

■ **STOP HORMONE THERAPY.** Estrogen and estrogen-progestin pills contribute to urinary incontinence by promoting the breakdown of collagen around the urethra, keeping it from closing. Stopping the pills can help with urinary incontinence.

Erectile Dysfunction

IT'S LATE AT NIGHT, the kids are in bed, and you and your partner are snuggled up on the couch, ready to pop in your favorite DVD. With the house so quiet, he gives you that familiar, mischievous grin, then leans over and nibbles on your ear (just where you like it). You wrap your arms around him and start to share in something you still always agree on after all these years: sex.

But this time, it's different. Something's wrong. He can't . . . *you know.*

He sweats . . . panics . . . makes excuses . . . apologizes. You worry: *Was it the wine with dinner? Or the long hours at work? The kids have been driving him crazy lately. . . .*

If this scenario rings too true, you and your partner are not alone. Erectile dysfunction (ED)—the persistent failure to achieve and/or maintain an erection sufficient for satisfactory sexual intercourse—affects up to 30 million men and their partners in the United States every year. And it's of particular concern for men with diabetes, who are up to three times more likely to have ED and develop the condition 10 to 15 years sooner than those without the disease. Chances are, if your partner has diabetes or prediabetes, there's more than stress behind his performance problems.

What's the Connection?

Achieving an erection requires a complex interplay of psychological, neurological, vascular, and hormonal factors, says Ira Sharlip, MD, FAUA, clinical professor of urology at the University of California, San Francisco, and spokesperson for the American Urological Association. When just one of these factors is off, a man may fail to achieve an erection. "While psychological factors are almost always involved, a man with diabetes usually suffers from vascular and neurological problems due to damaged blood vessels and nerves throughout the body," Dr. Sharlip says.

With a normal erection, a man becomes sexually aroused, either from direct sensory touch, stimulating visual images, or thoughts and feelings that elicit desire. His brain sends signals to his genitalia through neurotransmitters that travel to the corpora cavernosa—two cylindrical, spongelike chambers that span the length of the penile shaft. Each chamber contains a complex matrix of muscle (called smooth muscle), nerve and connective tissues, and arteries and veins that is protected by an expandable membrane called the tunica albuginea.

During arousal, neurotransmitter signals trigger smooth muscle relaxation. When this happens, the penile arteries expand and blood flows into the penis. Veins that normally drain blood out of the penis are compressed, or flattened, by the tunica albuginea. When blood is trapped, the penis becomes hard, erect, and ready for penetration.

In a man with diabetes, this process may be interrupted somewhere along the way, says Culley C. Carson III, MD, FAUA, chief of urology at the University of North Carolina at Chapel Hill and editor-in-chief of the medical journal *Contemporary Urology*. "The neurotransmitter primarily responsible for an erection, nitric oxide, may send signals to the smooth muscles; but if endothelial cells in the nerve endings of these muscles are damaged due to diabetic neuropathy, they will not respond," he says.

When the nervous system is intact, penile nerves produce more nitric oxide to help maintain the erection. However, if the body's vascular system is compromised due to heart disease or high blood pressure—as it so often is in men with diabetes—blood flow to the penile arteries is weakened or constricted, and the penis fails to become erect or stay hard long enough for sexual activity.

How Common Is It?

Think only women suffer from age-related hormonal changes? Men get them, too. Beginning in his 30s, a man's level of testosterone declines, causing a drop in libido and, sometimes, an inability to keep an erection. "Low testosterone is common in the diabetic population but has not been well publicized," says Dr. Carson, adding that this deficiency affects up to 30 percent of men with diabetes. "Patients will not only have lower sexual desire levels and less ability to sustain an erection throughout activity, but they will respond poorly to drugs used to treat ED."

Compounding the problem, sexual response time (from arousal to erection) lengthens as men age. The penis becomes less rigid due to decreased blood flow, and semen ejaculation during orgasm is less forceful and smaller in volume. Most men don't realize that these biological changes are a normal part of aging, says Barry McCarthy, PhD, ABPP, a clinical psychologist and sex therapist at American University in Washington, DC, who cowrote *Coping with Erectile Dysfunction: How to Regain Confidence and Enjoy Great Sex* and *Men's Sexual Health: Fitness for Satisfying Sex*. "At age 50, we can't run as fast as we did at 25—and we can't have the same sort of sexual responses, either," he says.

Let's face it: In early adulthood, all it takes is a slight breeze for a man to get an erection. Over the years, arousal becomes less spontaneous and predictable, but that doesn't mean that sex must be any less satisfying in middle age. "Men can still have great sex," Dr. McCarthy says. "They just need to move away from the notion of 'light-switch' sexuality—the perfunctory, automatic erections of youth—and move toward a deeper, more meaningful and mature idea of sex that includes a higher level of partner interaction and stimulation."

What Is His Risk?

While advancing age, hormonal changes, and neurological and vascular problems can trigger ED in a man with diabetes, additional health issues may also be to blame. If your partner has any of the following risk factors, his chances of ED are on the rise.

- Alcohol/drug abuse

- Cardiovascular disease, such as coronary artery disease and peripheral artery disease

- Depression or other mental health illness

- Hypertension

- High LDL (low-density lipoprotein) cholesterol—that's a reading of 160 mg/dL (milligrams per deciliter of blood) or higher

- Injury to the spinal cord or pelvic region

- Neurological disease such as multiple sclerosis, Alzheimer's disease, or Parkinson's disease

- Obesity or metabolic disorder

- Procedures for prostate cancer, including nerve-sparing prostatectomy and radiation

- Smoking

- Taking certain medications for high blood pressure, high cholesterol, depression, gastroesophageal reflux disease, or prostate cancer

- Uncontrolled blood glucose

If your partner has one or more of these risk factors, encourage him to talk to a physician. There's no surefire way to prevent ED, but acting on diabetes-related risk factors in his control—such as regulating blood sugar, quitting smoking, and losing weight—may help a man prevent the disorder or improve erectile function.

The Diabetes Lowdown

For many men, the diagnosis of ED brings news of another, larger problem to keep tabs on: coronary artery disease (CAD). In fact, the link between ED and CAD is so strong that many urologists refer patients directly to a cardiologist for a full workup or stress test before treating the sexual problem. "Studies show that men with erectile dysfunction have a much higher risk of having a cardiovascular event [such as a heart attack or stroke] within 3 to 5 years of the onset of their [ED] symptoms," says Culley C. Carson III, MD, FAUA, chief of urology at the University of North Carolina at Chapel Hill and editor-in-chief of the medical journal *Contemporary Urology*. "Unfortunately, erectile dysfunction is often a harbinger of things to come."

This may be especially true for men with diabetes. Even if they have no known cardiovascular risk factors, such as high cholesterol or hypertension, when they develop ED, they may be at an increased risk of developing heart disease. Italian researchers studying 133 men with diabetes found that uncomplicated cases had a "strong and independent association" between the presence of ED and subsequent CAD.

Because the penis requires large quantities of blood to produce an erection (even more than the heart needs to pump), it's often the first place that vascular disease shows up, Dr. Carson says. "Before erectile dysfunction can be treated, patients need to get their vascular risk factors under control," he says. "Recognizing this condition as an early warning sign of heart disease and seeing a cardiologist for treatment may not only help to improve a man's erectile function—it could save his life."

What Should I Watch For?

If your partner has performance problems, you'll notice. Urge him—lovingly—to seek help right away. Men who wait to seek treatment for ED or ignore the problem, hoping it will go away, suffer greater emotional hardships. "When men don't deal with their erectile problems, they begin to avoid sex completely because they want to prevent the pain and embarrassment of an awkward situation," says Stanley Althof, PhD, professor in the department of psychiatry and behavioral sciences at the University of Miami School of Medicine, professor in the department of urology at Case Western Reserve University, and executive director of the Center for Marital and Sexual Health of South Florida in West Palm Beach. "This leads to all sorts of problems within the relationship."

Men who stop initiating sex also stop activity that might lead to sex, such as holding hands, kissing, fondling, cuddling, or massage. Eliminating all forms of affectionate touch takes an emotional toll on a relationship. When they finally seek help for sexual dysfunction, couples who live more like siblings than lovers have twice as much work to do.

What Can We Do about It?

Erectile dysfunction isn't just "his" problem—it affects both of you. And working together, you can restore the most intimate part of your relationship. Start by establishing good communication both in and out of the bedroom, as well as exploring medical advice from a urologist.

Offer an Understanding Ear

Getting your partner to open up about ED won't be easy. He may feel ashamed, convinced that his problem makes him less of a man. He may get depressed, anxious, or irritable. He might even put the blame on you. But if you're prepared for this range of emotions, including the unfair fault-finding, you can better help your partner come to terms with his ED, says Dr. Althof. He offers this advice to women hoping to broach the topic with their mates.

■ **ARM YOURSELF WITH THE FACTS.** A man who understands that ED is a common complication of diabetes and a natural result of aging is less likely to ask "why me?" and more likely to accept the problem and find out ways to fix it.

■ **OFFER YOUR SUPPORT.** Listen to his concerns and fears. Let him know that you care, and offer to help in any way that you can. Focus on solutions, not on how ED is affecting your relationship.

■ **DON'T MAKE IT ABOUT YOU.** Avoid feeling sorry for yourself, and resist thinking that your partner is no longer attracted to you. Relax; it's not about you.

■ **BUILD HIS EGO.** Tell him you love him and enjoy having sex with him. Calm the irrational fear that men with ED sometimes have by assuring him that no, you don't want to sleep with another man: He's the one you want.

 When to See the Doctor

When ED begins to interfere with the majority of your sexual experiences as a couple, it's time for your partner to see a health care provider. Assure him that physicians who treat patients for diabetes are familiar with this complication, and brief him on what to expect.

During the evaluation, the physician will ask for your partner's medical and sexual history. Diagnostic tests may include a physical examination of the pelvic region, the genitalia, or the prostate; blood tests to check for low testosterone and high cholesterol and triglycerides; ultrasound imaging to assess the function of penile nerves and arteries; nerve function tests, such as squeezing the head of the penis to measure its response; and an NPTR (nocturnal penile tumescence and rigidity) test to determine if nocturnal erections occur during sleep.

If your partner shows signs of depression, anxiety, or another psychological problem, he may be referred to a therapist to help determine if any psychological or relationship issues may be affecting his erectile function. You might be asked to join him so you can discuss your own expectations of sexual activity.

Get Back in the Sack

Don't shy away from the bedroom. Difficulties during intercourse don't have to ruin a couple's sexual satisfaction at all, says Dr. McCarthy. "There are many things men and women can do to work around the problem of erectile dysfunction," he says. "The key to sexual fulfillment is to get creative." Next time you're in the mood, make these moves.

■ **BE THE AGGRESSOR.** Initiate sex yourself. There's nothing sexier to a man than a woman who wants him.

■ **GET PHYSICAL.** Sex is not a spectator sport—it requires team participation. Whip out that dusty old copy of *Kama Sutra* that you bought in the '70s for inspiration.

■ **ENGAGE IN ALL FORMS OF TOUCH.** Focus on physical exchanges that make both of you feel good.

■ **ALLEVIATE PERFORMANCE ANXIETY.** Don't make intercourse or even orgasm your end goal. Encourage your partner to think of you as a person with whom he enjoys intimacy and eroticism rather than someone for whom he must perform.

■ **TAKE A RAIN CHECK.** Scheduling a "pleasuring" date works well for many couples, Dr. McCarthy says. "Put a ban on intercourse for the night, and focus on pleasing each other," he suggests. "Light candles, take a bath together, listen to music, and have fun getting to know one another again through touch. You'd be surprised at how much this helps couples reconnect."

Explore Medical Options

Meanwhile, once a urologist has discussed therapeutic options for ED with your partner, sit down together and discuss the pros and cons of each choice. If you're fully committed to finding a strategy that works for both of you, the outlook is good, Dr. Sharlip says: "In a man dedicated to finding a cure, there's a 90 percent chance that he will be able to have satisfactory sexual function for the rest of his life."

A physician may recommend making lifestyle changes before exploring medical treatment. Your partner could decrease the incidence of ED by:

- Maintaining a healthy weight

- Eating a well-balanced diet approved by the American Diabetes Association

- Keeping blood glucose and hemoglobin A1C levels in check

- Lowering high blood pressure or cholesterol

- Exercising regularly

- Giving up smoking, recreational drugs, or excessive drinking

- Avoiding medications that cause erectile problems (your partner should ask his doctor whether ED could be a side effect of any medicines that he's taking)

- Engaging in psychological counseling or couples therapy

If erectile problems persist despite lifestyle changes, it's time for clinical measures. Below is a summary of treatments currently available for men with diabetes.

PHOSPHODIESTERASE (PDE) INHIBITORS: Sildenafil (Viagra), Vardenafil (Levitra), and tadalafil (Cialis) step up nitric oxide production to stimulate smooth muscles in the penis, allowing blood to flow into the corpora cavernosa. These oral drugs must be taken an hour before sexual activity and work only if a man is sexually aroused. A key caution: If a man takes nitroglycerin for chest pains or an alpha blocker for prostate enlargement or hypertension, PDE inhibitors are not recommended. They may cause a sudden—and deadly— drop in blood pressure. Also be aware that PDE inhibitors have a lower success rate for men with diabetes than in the general population. "About half of patients with diabetes find that these drugs don't work for them," Dr. Carson says. If a higher dose doesn't work, it's time to move on to other alternatives.

■ **TESTOSTERONE REPLACEMENT:** Men with lower-than-normal levels of testosterone might take oral or topical hormone replacement therapy (HRT), perhaps in combination with PDE inhibtors. In men, HRT doesn't carry the risks associated with treatment in women, such as cancer.

■ **INJECTION THERAPY:** Prior to sexual activity, the drug alprostadil is injected directly into the corpora cavernosa to expand penile arteries and increase blood flow. Results are quick—within 5 to 20 minutes of the shot—and the man needn't already be aroused to get an erection. It's effective for up to 75 percent of ED patients with diabetes. The downside: Side effects may include pain, swelling, or redness, or an erection that persists after orgasm.

■ **INTRAURETHRAL SUPPOSITORIES:** This offers a needle-free way to administer alprostadil or similar drugs used in injection therapy. Using an applicator, the man inserts a medicated tablet about 1 inch deep into the urethral canal. The tablet dissolves within 10 minutes, causing an erection that lasts from 30 to 60 minutes. Undesirable effects may include pain, redness, or a burning sensation, as well as minor urethral bleeding.

■ **VACUUM CONSTRICTION DEVICES:** Men who'd rather steer clear of shots and suppositories might try vacuum therapy. This less invasive treatment requires pumping to suck oxygen out of a plastic cylinder placed over the penile shaft. The vacuum effect draws blood into the penis and causes it to expand, creating an erection. An elastic band at the base of the penis constricts the blood supply and helps maintain the erection. This therapy works for up to 80 percent of men with diabetes.

■ **PENILE PROSTHESIS:** Though a last resort, this surgical treatment is effective in more than 90 percent of men. Two soft, hollow tubes are implanted into the corpora cavernosa, and a small pump is inserted into the scrotum. Activating the pump allows saline solution from a small balloon sac that's surgically implanted behind the abdominal wall to flow into the tubes, producing an erection. Once the sexual activity is over, the man pulls on a release valve in the scrotum, which releases fluid back into the balloon.

■ **HERBAL ANTIDOTES:** While there has been some anecdotal evidence of the benefits of herbal supplements such as ginseng, propionyl-L-carnitine, and

DHEA (dehydroepiandrosterone) in treating ED, there's no significant clinical research to back up any claims. Be aware, too, that herbal supplements are regulated as foods, not drugs, by the FDA, so they're not subject to the same standards of safety and effectiveness that medications are. One herb in particular, yohimbe—sometimes marketed as "herbal Viagra"—may cause adverse effects such as hypertension and heart failure and thus is not recommended for men with diabetes, who already are at increased risk for these conditions.

Become His Champion

Finding the right treatment for ED takes patience, resilience, and commitment on behalf of both partners. Unfortunately, dropout rates for treatments are high in patients with diabetes or other chronic diseases. Even when therapies work, men may give them up because of the inconvenience, side effects, or a loss of interest in sex due to depression or a troubled relationship. Work with your partner to help him overcome apprehensions about using erectile aids, and work to resolve difficulties within your marriage. Men whose women rally behind them fare much better during treatment for ED than those who don't have this support. Never let him settle for less, Dr. McCarthy says: "To be a good diabetic patient, one needs to address his overall health—and that includes sexual health. Giving up on sex is not the answer."

To find a board-certified urologist in your area, visit the American Urological Association's Web site at urologyhealth.org, or call 866-RING-AUA. Locate a certified sexuality educator, counselor, or therapist by logging on to the American Association of Sexualilty Educators, Counselors, and Therapists at aasect.org, or call 804-752-0026.

Peripheral Arterial Disease

CROW'S-FEET? Chalk it up to aging. Those wispy gray hairs? You can add those to the list. Reading glasses? No, they don't make you look like your mother, but yes—they are a consequence of age. Hot flashes? Just thank Father Time. Aches and pains? If you think those are also signs of aging, guess again.

Contrary to popular belief, aches and pains are not a normal part of aging. In fact, if you experience pain in your legs when you walk or even at rest, you could be suffering from a serious condition that increases your risk of cardio-vascular disease, heart attack, and stroke: peripheral arterial disease (PAD).

What's the Connection?

The "aching while active" phenomenon that occurs in PAD is really the hall-mark of the disease—and should be a red flag to physicians that something is wrong. In people with coronary artery disease (CAD), pain that occurs when the heart muscle is more active is called angina, or chest pain. In people with PAD, it's called claudication.

Claudication occurs when muscles in the legs, ankles, or feet fail to get the nutrients they need from the bloodstream. Activities that demand more energy—like walking, running, or climbing stairs—require muscles to absorb more oxygen and other elements from the blood in order to properly metabolize sugar into energy. But poor circulation, often due to a hardening of the arteries called atherosclerosis, limits blood flow to these areas. Arteries may be clogged with fat, cholesterol, calcium deposits, or other debris that, over time, narrow passageways and force blood to move more slowly through these areas. Severe blockages also can increase the risk of hypertension and lead to life-threatening thromboses (blood clots).

How Common Is It?

One out of every three people over the age of 50 who has diabetes has PAD. In the early stages, there are few symptoms of the disease—if any. Women are less likely to have symptoms (some studies say as many as 90 percent of women don't experience symptoms or have "unrecognized" symptoms of the disease), while those with diabetes are doubly challenged because diabetic neuropathy can reduce the capacity to feel any pain at all.

PAD symptoms you'll often feel are pain or cramping in the calves, thighs, or buttocks that becomes intense while walking or exercising but resolves within just a few minutes of rest. You won't be able to walk as far as you once used to—just taking a trip to the mailbox might be painful—and when you walk, you'll be slower.

What Is My Risk?

"Arteriosclerosis isn't discriminatory; it's an equal-opportunity offender," says Rear Admiral James M. Galloway, MD, FACP, FACC, Assistant Surgeon General and regional health administrator for the United States Public Health Service. He is also a cardiologist and associate professor of clinical and public health at the University Medical Center in Tucson. "When vascular disease presents in the legs, it's usually somewhere else, too," he says.

Consequently, PAD is a marker for vascular disease that involves the coronary, cerebral, or renal arteries. It puts you at a four to five times greater chance of someday having a heart attack or stroke. Consider that two out of three people with diabetes die from these or other heart disease–related events, and it's clear why an early diagnosis of PAD is important to avoid life-threatening implications.

Not surprisingly, risk factors for PAD are similar to risk factors for cardiovascular disease. Having diabetes or prediabetes already puts you at risk, but the following factors also increase your likelihood.

■ **SMOKING:** Next to diabetes, smoking is a leading cause of PAD. People who smoke are diagnosed with PAD an average of 10 years earlier than those who don't light up.

■ **UNCONTROLLED BLOOD SUGAR:** Elevated glucose levels above 100 to 125 mg/dL (milligrams per deciliter) put you at risk. High levels of the amino acid homocysteine in the blood pose an additional threat.

■ **OBESITY:** Weighing 30 percent or more than your ideal body weight puts a strain on vascular health.

■ **HIGH CHOLESTEROL:** Elevated "bad" LDL cholesterol and triglycerides increase plaque buildup in the arteries. A low level of "good" HDL cholesterol also ups your chances of vascular disease.

■ **HYPERTENSION:** Blood pressure above 130/80 mm Hg (millimeters of mercury) contributes to PAD.

■ **PHYSICAL INACTIVITY:** A sedentary lifestyle leads to obesity and other factors that put you at risk for vascular disease.

■ **GENDER:** Women are increasingly more likely to develop asymptomatic PAD as opposed to men, according to a 2007 study of data analyzed from 5,376 respondents to the National Health and Nutrition Examination Surveys.

■ **ETHNICITY:** African Americans and Latinos with diabetes are more likely than other minority groups to develop PAD.

■ **MEDICAL HISTORY:** A personal or family history of cardiovascular disease, heart attack, or stroke is highly associated with PAD.

■ **ADVANCING AGE:** People age 50 or older are more likely to develop vascular diseases like PAD.

When to See the Doctor

If the odds are stacked against you for PAD or you're suffering through painful claudication symptoms, it's time to see a doctor. Not all sources of leg pain—especially pain that appears during walking—are due to PAD. Spinal stenosis (a narrowing of the spinal cord), arthritis, a herniated disk, tarsal tunnel syndrome, or diabetic neuropathy can all cause similar pain. Only a health care provider can truly determine the source of your problem.

At the doctor's office, discuss your symptoms and include any history of vascular disease, smoking, or other factors that put you at risk for PAD. If you don't have symptoms, you should still be evaluated for the disease if you're age 50 or older and have diabetes, or if you're younger and have multiple cardiometabolic risk factors. Your physician should perform the following tests.

Blood pressure readings: Measurements should be taken in the arteries behind your knees and underneath your toes.

Ankle-brachial index (ABI): Comparing blood pressure measurements in your ankle to those in your arm may give physicians enough evidence to diagnose PAD. A significantly lower reading in the ankle is a hallmark of the disease.

Pulse checks: By placing a stethoscope over certain areas, health care providers can hear murmur-type sounds called bruits in the bloodstream, which indicate constricted areas of blood flow due to arterial blockages.

Physical examination: Checking your lower extremities helps to diagnose nonhealing wounds that could be markers for critical-limb ischemia. A 6-minute walking test evaluates symptoms of claudication. If you can't walk more than 2 miles per hour or a distance of 75 yards (the average length of one city block) without pain, you may have PAD.

Blood tests: High LDL cholesterol or triglycerides in the bloodstream could indicate vascular disease.

To confirm arteriosclerosis in your leg vessels, your physician may recommend additional testing, such as ultrasound, MRI (magnetic resonance imaging), or CT (computed tomography) scanning. At the same time, schedule cardiovascular screening tests to evaluate the presence of arteriosclerosis in the coronary arteries that lead to the heart or the carotid arteries that lead to the brain.

Unfortunately, most people with vascular disease have not just one but multiple risk factors. For example, if you have diabetes, you are more likely to also have high cholesterol or excess weight gain, compared with someone without diabetes. This strong association between risk factors is called your cardiometabolic risk. The more risk factors that you have, the higher

RESEARCH BUZZ

Get "FITT"

To help you gain the best results from walking, your physician may recommend you participate in a supervised walking program at a cardiac gym or other medical facility. It may be difficult to find a program nearby, however, and medical insurance often doesn't cover the training, so few people get to participate in these programs.

As a result, Mary McGrae McDermott, MD, associate professor of medicine in the department of medicine at Northwestern University Feinberg School of Medicine, set out to determine whether following a self-directed walking program would provide equal benefit. Results from her 2006 study on 417 people found independent walking to be "a rational alternative" to supervised walking for preventing the functional decline of walking in patients with PAD. "We found that people who went walking for exercise at least three times a week for a total of 90 minutes or more had significantly slower rates of decline in their walking performance, compared with the PAD patients who didn't walk for exercise at all or those who walked for exercise only once or twice a week," Dr. McDermott says.

So walking on your own can be a viable alternative to training in a cardiac gym—if you follow the proper protocol. "The key is to walk at the right intensity," says Michael Crawford, an exercise physiologist at the Cleveland Clinic's Preventive Cardiology Clinic. "If it doesn't hurt, you're not going to reap the benefits. This is the only time a health care provider will tell you 'no pain, no gain.'"

He recommends that patients follow the FITT model of exercise, which stands for frequency of exercise, intensity of activity, type of exercise, and time or duration of activity. You can participate in your cardiometabolic risk index—and the more likely you are to develop other complications that increase your likelihood of PAD, CAD, a heart attack, or stroke.

this program at home or in a gym by adhering to the guidelines below.

Frequency: Walk at least three times a week, with a goal of five times per week.

Intensity: Pain should begin to set in after 3 to 5 minutes of walking and become severe after 5 to 10 minutes. If you don't feel pain, you're probably not walking fast enough. Increase your speed, or walk on an incline to reach the intensity you need. If you're walking on a treadmill, set your speed to between 1 to 3 miles per hour (find a speed that allows you to walk about 10 minutes before having to stop). If you can walk faster than 3 miles per hour on the treadmill, add up to 5 percent of elevation to get the intensity you need. Once you reach a point where claudication pain is too intense, stop. Find a nearby seat and rest for a few minutes. The pain should resolve within a few minutes, and then you can start walking again.

Type: Walking—it trains the leg muscles to do more with less better than any other type of activity.

Time: Walk at least 30 minutes at a time, with a goal of reaching 50 minutes. Remember that you will have to allot more time for each walking session because you will need to stop periodically. For example, if you can walk only 5 minutes at a time, you will need to perform six intervals to reach a total of 30 minutes of movement. This may take you an hour to complete.

Before starting your new walking program, consult your physician. Once you begin, don't expect to notice any improvement in your walking ability for at least 3 months. If you want to see how well you've progressed in the meantime, go back to your former walking intensity. You'll be surprised to find you're able to walk at that pace for 10, 20, 30, or even 50 minutes without needing to rest.

What Should I Watch For?

In people who have diabetes or prediabetes, PAD usually strikes the lower leg between the knee and foot. This tends to be where arteries are significantly blocked and would explain why most circulation problems are concentrated in the ankle or foot. Physicians can't say for sure why this part of the leg is affected most. Likewise, they can't pinpoint exactly why a person with arteriosclerosis develops symptoms in their legs first, instead of, say, the coronary arteries. But one thing is clear: If you have PAD, chances are other vascular areas in your body are affected. The symptoms just haven't shown up—yet.

When you don't manage arteriosclerosis through diet, exercise, or medication, symptoms of claudication become worse. Pain that usually resolves during restful activities—like watching television—can linger for hours or days. If blood flow is significantly compromised, you may develop critical-limb ischemia, occlusion of leg arteries that causes slow-healing foot ulcers; foot deformities, such as hammertoes and bunions; or numbness, tingling, or coldness in the lower extremities. Skin may lose its healthy glow and become dry or cracked. In the most severe cases of critical-limb ischemia, gangrene may develop. When this happens, an amputation is necessary to preserve surrounding tissue.

What Can I Do about It?

If you're diagnosed with PAD, there's a lot you can do to reduce the painful symptoms of claudication, increase your ability to ambulate freely, and even significantly reduce your risk factors for other types of cardiovascular disease.

■ **GET BLOOD SUGAR LEVELS IN CHECK.** Your A1C level should be less than 7. If it's not, talk to your endocrinologist about medications to help control your blood sugar. If you're a smoker, set a quit date and stick to it. You may have tried quitting before, so you know it's not easy. But today there are many

The Diabetes Lowdown

Quitting smoking? Taking new cholesterol-lowering medications? Adding a walking program to your exercise schedule? See how these changes make a big difference in your health by logging on to the American Diabetes Association's Diabetes PHD (Personal Health Decisions) risk assessment tool at diabetes.org/phd/profile/default.jsp. You'll get a personalized assessment of your current risk factors for different conditions, such as heart attack, stroke, kidney failure, or eye disease. Add new information about the lifestyle changes you plan to make, and you'll see how well these modifications will affect your future health.

Before logging on, be sure to have the following information at hand. You'll be asked for it when you create your personal profile.

- Basic personal information (such as age, weight, gender)

- Health history (including whether you smoke, are physically active, or have undergone health-related events such as a heart attack or stroke)

- Basic family health history (including incidence of diabetes or heart disease)

- Blood pressure levels

- Cholesterol levels

- Fasting glucose level A1C

- Current medications related to diabetes, blood pressure, or cholesterol

To learn more about the Diabetes PHD tool, log on to the ADA at diabetes.org.

options—such as patches and other tools—to help you kick the habit (see Smoking on page 206).

■ **TAKE IT A DAY AT A TIME.** Your physician may also suggest that you lose weight and lower your cholesterol or blood pressure through diet and exercise. That usually means more fresh fruits, vegetables, whole grains, and legumes and less highly processed carbohydrates, trans fats, and saturated fats—which may be drastically different from your usual menu. And if you're new to exercise, doing an all-new activity might be daunting. In fact, most people feel so overwhelmed by these changes that they quit before they start, Dr. Galloway says. "Patients view these lifestyle modifications as too challenging, so they just give up," he says. "What people need to hear is that just making one or two small changes each day, and then building upon that, will add up to major differences in your health."

■ **MAKE MINOR MENU MODIFICATIONS.** Starting tomorrow, change the habit that's easiest to modify. If you eat cereal every morning, add strawberries, blueberries, or bananas to get the day's first serving of fruits. If you're too rushed for a proper breakfast, grab a banana or orange when you're heading out the door, and eat another piece of fruit for an afternoon snack. It will make you feel much better than that leftover piece of cake from the office birthday party.

Here are more heart-healthy choices to incorporate into your everyday diet. Some are so easy, you won't even realize you're doing something good!

SWAP OUT	ADD IN	WHY IT'S A BETTER CHOICE
Whole or 2% milk	Fat-free or 1% milk	Less fat, saturated fat, and cholesterol
Table salt	Sodium-free spices such as Mrs. Dash	Less sodium but packs just as much flavor
Cheese	Low-fat cheese	Less fat, saturated fat, and cholesterol
Fruit juice	Whole fruit	Less sugar, more fiber
Ice cream	Frozen yogurt, low-fat ice cream	Less fat
Butter	Extra virgin olive oil	Less fat, cholesterol
Egg yolks	Egg whites, egg substitutes	Less cholesterol
White bread	Whole grain, multigrain, enriched white bread	Less fat, trans fat, and sugar; more fiber

(Source: American Diabetes Association)

■ **ADD MEDICATION TO THE MIX.** In conjunction with a healthy diet, certain medications may help reduce cholesterol, blood pressure, and your chance of stroke. They include statins for high LDL cholesterol, ACE inhibitors for abnormal blood pressure levels, and anti-thrombotic drugs such as aspirin to help prevent blood clots. In fact, taking between 75 to 162 milligrams daily of over-the-counter aspirin has been shown to prevent blood clots that lead to stroke. Before beginning any new medication, consult your physician.

■ **TIE ON YOUR WALKING SHOES.** "Walking is one of the best therapies for peripheral arterial disease," says Michael Crawford, an exercise physiologist at the Cleveland Clinic's Preventive Cardiology Clinic. He also runs the center's PAD rehabilitation program. "A structured walking program can improve walking ability between 100 to 150 percent—more than any surgical procedure for PAD can offer. What's more, you get all the cardiovascular benefits, like improved muscle tone; lower blood sugar, cholesterol, and blood pressure; and calorie burning to help you lose weight."

The PAD prescription: Walk for exercise for 30 minutes or more at least three times a week. For minor to moderate symptoms of claudication, this schedule may increase your overall walking ability better than any traditional procedure for PAD. The question you may be asking, however, is: *How can I walk if I'm in pain?*

"The key is to walk for only a few minutes at a time—until the pain becomes severe," Crawford says. "Stop and rest for a few minutes. Then start up again. You may have to stop and start several times over the course of your walk, but the longer you do this, the more you'll be able to walk further without pain."

Treating Limb-Threatening Ischemia

If debilitating pain due to critical-limb ischemia is plaguing you, walking even short distances may be difficult or impossible. Your physician may prescribe cilostazol or pentoxifylline, two medications that ease claudication symptoms and may even improve walking ability. But if pain becomes too intense or poor circulation causes slow-healing foot ulcers, you may need surgery. The following surgical procedures help improve blood flow to the ankles and feet.

■ **ANGIOPLASTY:** A small catheter is inserted into the femoral artery, and a tiny balloon is fed through this device. The balloon is then inflated inside the artery to widen it and crush blockages. To help keep the pathway open, a small, cylindrical mesh stent is inserted into the artery.

■ **REVASCULARIZATION (BYPASS SURGERY):** Blood flow in the leg is rerouted around blockages in the femoral artery. Surgeons use a portion of your own healthy vein to circumvent the blockage or place a man-made synthetic tube above and below the damaged pathway to improve circulation.

After surgery, your walking performance may improve, but beginning a structured program will help you walk further, faster, and for longer periods of time. Exercise training also helps to reduce inflammation in arterial walls and improve endothelial function, which causes blood vessels to dilate so that more blood can get to where it's needed. It may also promote the growth of new blood vessels in the legs.

Foot Complications

YOUR FEET MAY NOT BE particularly glamorous, but they deserve top billing in your diabetes care. Neglected feet could otherwise lead to some of the most devastating effects of the disease: slow-healing wounds, infection, and even limb loss.

"Foot problems are the number one reason people with diabetes end up in the hospital," says Crystal Holmes, DPM, instructor of podiatry at the University of Michigan department of internal medicine and spokesperson for the American Podiatric Medical Association. "Strictly managing your glucose, reducing your risk factors for heart disease, and protecting and pampering your feet are key to keeping them healthy."

What's the Connection?

With 26 bones; 33 joints; more than 100 muscles, ligaments, and tendons working in synergy; and an intricate network of nerves and blood vessels, the human foot is a complex structure. Consequently, there's lots of room for error, especially if you have diabetes. If high blood sugar damages nerves and arteries throughout the body, the feet can really take a beating.

■ **NEUROPATHY:** Another word for nerve damage, neuropathy affects a majority of people with diabetes. The longer you have the disease, the more likely you are to develop nerve damage. The condition progresses slowly, beginning with reduced feeling in your foot. You might find yourself unable to feel light touch or vibration or differentiate between hot and cold. Nerves stop sending signals to the skin to maintain itself, so sweat glands fail to produce moisture and oil, and the skin becomes dry and flaky. Neuropathy may also cause abnormal sensations such as pins-and-needles tingling; burning, shooting pain; or numbness. (We'll talk more about nerve damage on page 125.)

■ **DIABETIC ULCERS:** These sores can stem from any sort of trauma, including some seemingly minor nuisances: walking barefoot, wearing ill-fitting shoes, stubbing your toe, and having ingrown toenails or dry, cracked feet. Any of these can put you at risk for a diabetic ulcer—an open wound that's slow to heal. "If you're unable to feel pain in a normal way, you're unable to feel a pebble in your shoe—and you'll continue to walk on it," Dr. Holmes says. When you keep applying pressure to the affected area because you're literally numb to the problem, the healing process is interrupted.

■ **PERIPHERAL ARTERIAL DISEASE (PAD):** If you've ever been awakened in the middle of the night by pain in your feet, legs, or thighs or all the way up to your buttocks, you may have PAD, a vascular disease that inhibits blood flow. Diabetes is a leading risk factor for PAD (so is smoking), according to Peter Sheehan, MD, professor of endocrinology at Mount Sinai School of Medicine, director of the Diabetes Center of Greater New York at Cabrini Medical Center, and a spokesperson for the American Diabetes Association. "A buildup of cholesterol and plaque can cause a blockage or narrowing of the arteries that supply blood to the legs," he says. "While symptoms are not always present, patients may feel pain that stops during rest. They also might feel like they can't walk as fast as they used to because their legs feel heavy or tired."

PAD also slows circulation and, thus, healing of diabetic foot ulcers. Less blood is available to carry oxygen and nutrients to the wound site, inhibiting the body's ability to fight off bacteria that enter the wound. Instead, they multiply, causing an infection that tunnels down through the skin and into underlying tissue, bone, and joints. Untreated, this could lead to a serious bone infection or blood flow problems and contribute to gangrene, a deadening of tissue that will require amputation. Once you have an amputation, your chances of needing another one rise dramatically. The key word here is *untreated*. Remember, almost all of these amputations are preventable—meaning the fate of your feet lies in your hands.

How Common Is It?

If you allow cuts, sores, infections, or pains in your foot to go untreated or undiagnosed, you could end up losing a toe—or even your whole foot—to surgery for the sake of preserving the rest of your limb. In fact, as many as 86,000 lower limbs are amputated each year due to diabetes-related complications.

But there's good news—95 percent of amputations are avoidable through preventive care. Regular TLC for your tootsies will also help you avoid more severe forms of neuropathy that weaken the muscles and bones that support the foot, leading to painful deformities such as hammertoes that curl under the feet. The metatarsal heads of toes (the "knuckles") subsequently drop down and grind against the floor. Weak muscles also may cause the big toe to point inward toward the smaller toes and develop a bony prominence, or bunion, at its joint. Deformities like these increase the risk of corns, calluses, blisters, and open sores as the foot rubs against shoes and other flat surfaces, as well as contribute to balance problems and arthritis.

A much more serious deformity affecting people with diabetes who have nerve damage is Charcot arthropathy, or Charcot foot. This rare condition softens bones and weakens muscles, raising the risk for bone fractures, sprained ankles, and, eventually, collapsed arches. Fortunately, if you heed early warning signs, such as redness and swelling, you can get treated and avoid permanent deformities that can only be corrected with surgery and physical therapy.

What Is My Risk?

Awareness is your best defense. To find out if you're at risk of foot ulcers due to nerve or circulation problems, ask your podiatrist to perform the following quick, painless, and noninvasive tests at least once a year.

■ **FOOT EXAMINATION:** Your feet should be checked for problems such as deep cuts, sores, rashes, infections, and structural deformities. Corns and calluses (thick layers of skin caused by too much pressure) can irritate healthy skin underneath, posing a risk for infection. Bacteria can also enter the body through cracked skin that splits and bleeds or toenails that lift up from the nail bed.

■ **MONOFILAMENT TEST:** This simple exam can be performed within seconds. A health care provider taps a small nylon wire resembling fishing line against various locations on the sole of your foot. If you can't feel the sensations the majority of the time, that signals neuropathy.

■ **VIBRATION PERCEPTION THRESHOLD (VPT):** A forklike device called a biothesiometer applies small vibrations to the padding of the big toe. If you can't feel it, you may have neuropathy.

■ **ANKLE-BRACHIAL INDEX (ABI):** By checking the blood pressure in your ankles, legs, and feet and comparing those numbers with the blood pressure in your arm, your physician can look for decreased blood flow or PAD. If blood pressure is low, you may need Doppler ultrasound testing, which uses sound waves to measure blood flow in the feet and legs.

During your consultation, tell your physician if you notice hair loss, hot or cold spots, or pulsating areas in your foot, which may indicate poor circulation. Also mention if you're experiencing tingling or numbness, which are signs of neuropathy.

What Should I Watch For?

Each day, before putting on your socks and shoes, inspect your feet, starting with the soles. Then move on to your toes, toenails, between your toes, arches, heels, and the tops of your feet. If you have vision problems due to diabetic neuropathy or another eye disease, enlist a family member to help check your feet. A mirror may also be useful to view hard-to-see areas. Be sure to look for signs of discoloration, "pulsating" or warm spots, dryness, lodged objects that you can't feel due to neuropathy, and any other change in the structure or appearance of your feet. If you have a history of diabetic ulcers, checking your feet twice a day (at night and in the morning) is recommended.

If you notice swelling, redness, or hot spots, ask your physician to check for Charcot foot. Many health care providers mistake the signs of this condition for skin inflammation, so be specific about your concern.

What Can I Do about It?

The best way to sidestep foot problems is to get your diabetes under control. That means you should:

- Know how and when to test your blood sugar levels.

- Have A1C and cholesterol levels checked regularly.

- Take medications as prescribed by your physician.

- Eat a well-balanced diet that includes low-fat, high-fiber foods.

- Stop smoking—tobacco inhibits circulation.

- Refrain from alcohol abuse, which can worsen the effects of neuropathy.

- Exercise regularly to improve circulation in your legs.

- Practice daily foot care.

That last step might just be the easiest part of being a good diabetes patient. All that's required is soap, water, and a little common sense.

Everyday TLC

To start, wash your feet every day with lukewarm water and a mild, non-irritating soap. Pat your feet dry, paying special attention to the webbed areas between your toes, where moisture could lead to fungal infections. Since dry, cracked skin is also a pathway for infection, be sure to moisturize your feet with a cream or lotion after drying them. When purchasing over-the-counter (OTC) products, look for those that bear the seal of approval from the American Podiatric Medical Association. Skin softeners that help keep skin supple while reducing the incidence of corns and calluses include Keralac and AmLactin.

If you have a history of fungal infections, consider applying an antifungal gel, cream, or powder. Medicated powders reduce sweating and help prevent a damp environment within your shoe, which is the ideal breeding ground for fungi, bacteria, and viruses.

RESEARCH BUZZ

Got Heat?

Taking your daily foot temperature with a handheld foot thermometer can alert you to early warning signs of infection, according to a study of 173 diabetes patients at Texas A&M Health Science Center.

In the multicenter trial, those with a history of foot ulcers were given information on prevention and trained to properly examine their feet. Patients were told to contact a nurse at the first sign of redness, hot spots, or inflammation. One group also received an infrared skin thermometer to check for a rise in temperature—a sign of infection. These patients were told that if their foot temperatures increased, they should contact a nurse immediately, reduce their activity, and take fewer steps on the affected foot until temperature readings returned to normal.

The researchers found that patients who received only educational materials and conducted foot exams were four times more likely to develop foot ulcers than those aided by foot thermometers. Digital thermometers are available with a doctor's prescription and cost about $150.

At-Home Rx

Knowing how to properly care for your feet when you notice problems will help keep you from needing treatment at the doctor's office—or the hospital. Below are tips for dealing with (and preventing) common foot-related problems.

Note: Be sure to consult your physician before starting any home-care regimen. Corns and warts often look alike, and athlete's foot can also resemble cellulitis, a dangerous bacterial skin infection, so it's important to get a professional opinion before treating the problem yourself.

■ **ATHLETE'S FOOT:** This red, rashlike fungal infection appears on or around toes. Regularly using topical OTC antifungal agents will help to treat and prevent further infections. Spraying the insides of your shoes with an antibacterial spray can also help kill fungus and bacteria. If OTCs don't cure your case, your physician may prescribe a stronger medication.

■ **BUNIONS:** Unless this joint deformity is infected, painful, or swollen, there's no need for surgery or physical therapy. Just wear shoes that are wide enough to accommodate the ball of your foot so you prevent corns or calluses from forming on your bunion. Cushioning the area with OTC pads can also provide relief.

■ **CORNS/CALLUSES:** If you don't have a condition that inhibits wound healing, use a pumice stone to file down these areas of thickened skin. (Never use razors or clippers to remove dead skin as applying too much pressure can cause an open wound.) Do this right after bathing, when your skin is softer and easier to manage. Skip OTC corn or callus removers because these products contain salicylic acid, which eats away at healthy skin. If you have neuropathy, poor circulation, or PAD, don't treat corns or calluses yourself. Your physician can safely excise dead skin cells manually using a scalpel.

■ **FUNGAL NAILS:** Thick, brittle, yellowed, or disfigured nails signal a fungal infection below. An OTC topical treatment such as a clear nail polish applied to the top of the nail may be enough to cure the infection. Consult your physician if the problem persists despite OTC treatment.

■ **HAMMERTOES:** Toes that curl under can put you at risk for corns and calluses. To avoid friction from your socks, wear low-heeled shoes with deep toe boxes. A pad that attaches directly to the toes may also reduce rubbing. If your hammertoes hurt or cause trouble with walking, ask your physician about surgical treatments to release the tendons or remove pieces of bone. Physical therapy may also help straighten toes.

■ **INGROWN TOENAILS:** Nails that grow downward into the skin can cause painful sores that lead to infection. Prevent the problem by cutting your toenails straight across and not too far down—they should be no shorter than the end of your toe. If you have an ingrown toenail, don't treat it yourself. See a physician.

■ **PLANTAR WARTS:** When viruses burrow into your skin, they form a tiny, calluslike barrier for protection. This is a wart. Most warts are painless and go away on their own. If you have one that causes discomfort, treat it with an OTC wart remover if your immune system is not compromised by poor circulation or PAD and you don't have neuropathy.

Wound Care

If you find a superficial cut or scrape on your foot, clean it with lukewarm water and a mild soap, then apply a topical antibiotic cream. Never use harsh chemicals such as peroxide or alcohol, which can destroy healthy skin cells needed for healing. Cover the wound with a bandage. Within 24 to 48 hours, the wound should begin to form a scab, which will become darker and thicker with time. If your sore does not form a scab, drains excessively, or becomes very red, call your podiatrist immediately. A small cut can turn quickly into a very serious wound infection.

Finding a deeper cut that bleeds is also cause for action. Visit a health care provider within 24 to 48 hours of discovering an open cut, sore, or blister on your foot. In the past you might have relied on your body's natural healing process, but diabetes may be compromising your body's traditional response to wounds, so now you're going to need some extra help.

Medical treatment begins with a thorough cleaning using topical enzymes to break down dead tissue or surgical excision to cut it away. Vacuum drainage devices remove excess fluid. This wound cleaning, or debridement, creates a disease-free environment that is optimal for healing.

If you have an infection, topical, oral, or intravenous antibiotics may be prescribed. To jump-start the healing process, medications are applied directly to the wound, and—if that's not enough—advanced therapies such as hyperbaric oxygen therapy, which increases oxygen in the blood, may be enlisted. If it's a large wound, a surgeon may place a bioengineered skin graft over the site, covering it with a bandage to prevent bacteria from entering.

Continuing to walk on a wound will slow healing and may cause an infection to tunnel up into the muscles and bones of your feet, so you may need to wear an orthotic cast or shoe insert. Your podiatrist will measure you for one of these custom-fitted devices to take the pressure off wounds on the bottom or sides of your feet.

During diagnosis or treatment, your physician may determine that slow healing or a serious wound infection is the result of PAD. You may then be referred to a vascular surgeon for further testing or surgical treatment to open up blocked arteries in your legs.

Avoiding Future Problems

After treatment for a diabetic ulcer, you'll want to avoid the problem that put you in the doctor's office in the first place. Friction from a poorly fitting shoe is the number one cause of corns, calluses, and open sores that lead to diabetic ulcers. Wearing comfortable—and safe—shoes is imperative. And can you think of a better excuse to go shoe shopping?

Your new shoes may be covered under the *Medicare Therapeutic Shoe Bill*. This bill was enacted by Congress to provide proper footwear and inserts for people with diabetes at high risk for ulcers and amputations from conditions such as neuropathy and vascular disease. The benefit permits you to get one pair of shoes (including roomier "extra-depth" shoes or custom-molded ones), inserts, and/or shoe modifications each year. To find out if you qualify, contact your podiatrist.

The Diabetes Lowdown

Having diabetes doesn't mean you can never wear cute pumps or dressy heels or pamper yourself with a pedicure. You just need to put in a little extra thought and care.

Regarding heels: "If you don't have a history of balance problems or weak ankles, wearing a heel height of 2 inches or under won't have a detrimental effect on your feet," says Crystal Holmes, DPM, instructor of podiatry at the University of Michigan department of medicine and spokesperson for the American Podiatric Medical Association. "But wearing heels higher than that will jam toes in the toe box, crushing hammertoes and bunions, and increase the amount of pressure on your foot sevenfold."

If you enjoy wearing heels, change it up. Wear flats and heels of different heights each day so your tendons don't become inflamed. Before slipping into shoes, check them for loose objects such as pebbles, stones, and even small insects that may be hiding out. You'd be surprised at what can get into your shoe after a day of walking, working out in the yard, or just hanging around the house.

Before scheduling a pedicure, check with your podiatrist. If you have neuropathy, circulation problems, or certain skin infections, you won't want to entrust your feet to someone who's not a medical professional.

Once you get the green light, find a salon that adheres to strict safety regulations and has never violated health codes. Call the salon directly and ask for this information (which is in the public domain), or contact your local Better Business Bureau. It's possible to contract fungal infections, cellulitis, and even hepatitis from unsterilized instruments at nail salons. To protect yourself, only frequent salons with single-use, disposable instruments. You might also bring your own instruments from a nail kit, which you can buy at most superstores or pharmacies. To kill bacteria, wipe your manicure tools with alcohol after every use. Never get your cuticles cut, and avoid exfoliating or shaving your legs before getting a pedicure. Cuts and microderm abrasions provide an excellent pathway for germs to enter the body.

Before choosing the perfect shoes, you'll need to adopt some shoe smarts. Follow these tips when out and about.

- Purchase shoes at the end of the day, when your feet are swollen.

- Get measured (foot sizes change over time).

- Steer clear of pointy or open-toe shoes, strappy sandals, or thongs that put undue pressure on different areas of your feet.

- Avoid vinyl or plastic shoes that don't let your feet breathe.

- Stick to soft microfiber socks that wick away moisture.

- Avoid socks with thick seams if you have neuropathy.

- Try on both the left and right shoe of a possible pair with the socks you intend to wear.

- Be sure each shoe provides enough room for your longest toe (which may be the second or third toe) and the widest part of your feet.

- Don't buy shoes that are more than a half an inch longer than your feet.

- Don't settle for less than perfect fit. If shoes don't feel good in the store, they won't feel good at home.

- Break in new shoes slowly, wearing them for no longer than an hour a day.

Learning to take good care of your feet can be a process of trial and error. Being a vigilant diabetes patient is no easy feat—so to speak—but following the above guidelines will help keep your toes in tip-top shape.

Hypoglycemia

CONSIDERING THAT MOST of the problems and complications of diabetes stem from *high* blood sugar levels, it may seem contradictory at first that hypoglycemia, or *low* blood sugar, is also linked to diabetes. As anyone with diabetes will tell you, though, the disease is about more than just preventing spiked blood sugar—it's about keeping it as close to balanced as you can at all times. That level is precarious at best—just as some factors can make blood sugar rocket upward, others can send it tumbling down.

What's the Connection?

A number of things can lead to hypoglycemia. "Hypoglycemia generally occurs in people with diabetes when there is an imbalance between intake of food fuels and their use in the individual's body," says Gabriel I. Uwaifo, MD, associate professor of endocrinology in the department of medicine at the University of Mississippi in Jackson. "Since many people with diabetes take medicines to lower blood glucose, hypoglycemia tends to occur when there is an imbalance between caloric intake and the use of medications. Such imbalances could be based on timing or mismatches in the amount of food and medication." Dr. Uwaifo adds that other common scenarios include:

- Exercising vigorously without eating or eating too little

- Exercising vigorously while taking diabetes medicine

- Taking too much diabetes medicine

- Drinking too much alcohol, especially when paired with diabetes medication and/or not enough food

- Taking diabetes medicine along with other drugs that increase hypoglycemia risk, such as beta-blockers

- Taking diabetes medicine without first checking blood glucose levels

How Common Is It?

Almost everyone with diabetes will experience low blood sugar at one point or another. And the severity and frequency of the episodes will vary quite a bit based on a number of health factors, as well as the number of times you experience the situations mentioned above.

Although those with type 1 diabetes are more likely to experience hypoglycemia than those with the more common type 2, it's a risk factor in both conditions. "In type 1 diabetes, the pancreas does not produce insulin, so type 1 diabetics must inject insulin to survive," says Beverly Caskey, RPh, a Medco pharmacist who specializes in diabetes care. "Too much insulin, and the patient experiences low blood sugar, but not enough insulin, and the patient will have blood sugar that is too high. Many type 2 diabetics are able to control blood sugar with oral medications that are less likely to cause episodes of hypoglycemia."

As a result, adds Dr. Uwaifo, rates of hypoglycemia hover around 16 to 20 percent for type 2 patients on oral medication, 30 to 50 percent for type 2 patients on insulin, and close to 100 percent for people with type 1 diabetes.

It's also worth noting that hypoglycemia is fairly uncommon in the general population, says David L. Katz, MD, MPH, director of the Yale Prevention Research Center in Derby, Connecticut, and author of *The Way to Eat*. "A lot of people may feel fatigued and think they have low blood sugar, but they really don't," he says. "A blood test is needed to determine whether or not someone is experiencing hypoglycemia."

What Is My Risk?

Though hypoglycemia is often misidentified in the general population, the implications of the condition can be quite serious for those who experience it. That's why people—particularly those with diabetes—need to be aware of the symptoms and treat it as an emergency if it occurs. To help you assess your own risk of hypoglycemia, Dr. Uwaifo has come up with the following questions.

- Do you have type 1 diabetes?

- Do you use insulin?

- Do you use sulphonylureas (medicines such as glipizide and glimepiride) or meglitinides (such as nateglinide or repaglinide) to help control glucose?

- Do you drink alcohol regularly (daily or more than once a day)?

- Do you exercise for 30 minutes or more at least three times a week?

- Have you had low blood glucose levels (less than 50 mg/dL, or milligrams per deciliter) that you discovered by checking your levels at home in the last 3 months, but you exhibited no symptoms?

- Do you frequently wake up drenched in sweat during the night or early in the morning?

According to Dr. Uwaifo, answering yes to one to three questions suggests a moderate risk of hypoglycemia, and four or more affirmatives signal a severe risk. "Such persons should check their blood glucose more frequently than they presently do and consider instituting other preventive measures," he says. "A discussion with a health care provider would also be worthwhile."

What Should I Watch For?

Mention of low blood sugar may evoke thoughts of fatigue, weakness, and other minor symptoms that can be cured with a drink of juice or a few pieces of candy. But Caskey warns against taking such a laid-back approach. "Hypoglycemia can be dangerous or even life-threatening, depending on the level, duration, and where the event occurs. It should be treated as a medical emergency," she says. "Severe, sustained low blood sugar can even result in loss of consciousness or death."

Thankfully, the symptoms of hypoglycemia are usually pretty apparent and easy to spot. (The one frightening exception to this is hypoglycemia unawareness; see "The Diabetes Lowdown" on page 123.) And they often arrive in stages that progressively worsen, so you'll know how serious the condition is based on your symptoms. Here's what to look for.

☤ When to See the Doctor

- If you have diabetes, ask your doctor about the risks of hypoglycemia and how they apply to your case, how you can best handle an episode, and how to obtain emergency medicine (such as glucagon) if necessary.

- If you experience early-stage symptoms (anxiety, hunger, heart palpitations, profuse sweating, rapid breathing, or tiredness) for the first time, see your doctor to confirm that you have hypoglycemia and need treatment.

- If symptoms persist or worsen despite multiple carbohydrate or glucagon treatments, seek emergency medical care immediately.

EARLY-STAGE SYMPTOMS

- Anxiety
- Hunger
- Heart palpitations
- Profuse sweating
- Rapid breathing
- Tiredness

MIDDLE-STAGE SYMPTOMS

- Increasing drowsiness and fatigue
- Weakness
- Confusion
- Blurred vision
- Difficulty concentrating and poor memory
- Change in personality and unusual behavior
- Poor performance with tasks requiring hand-eye coordination (such as reading, writing, or driving)

LATE-STAGE SYMPTOMS

- Loss of consciousness
- Seizures
- Nerve and/or brain damage

As you might have guessed, the urgency of treatment increases with the severity of these symptoms, as discussed below.

What Can I Do about It?

Hypoglycemia is usually easy to treat if detected early enough. Below, we'll first outline the steps required to end an active case, and then offer a few strategies for preventing it in the future.

■ **PRACTICE THE RULE OF 15S.** Caskey says the "Rule of 15s" offers an easy way to remember how to properly treat hypoglycemia. When you feel hypoglycemia kicking in (or see a loved one experiencing it), treat it with 15 grams of carbohydrates. Then wait 15 minutes, check blood glucose levels, and take in (or administer) another 15 grams of carbs if blood sugar is still too low. "Some examples of 15 grams of carbohydrates are 3 to 4 ounces of juice, 4 ounces of regular soda, 2 teaspoons of sugar, or 3 to 5 glucose tablets," she says.

■ **HAVE GLUCAGON ON HAND.** In more serious cases, in which the person is too lethargic or confused to take anything orally, someone will need to administer glucagon, which is an intramuscular injection. For this reason, people prone to hypoglycemia need to have glucagon on hand at all times, as

---

RESEARCH BUZZ ....

Kinder, Gentler Glucose Monitoring

For many people with diabetes, one of the keys to preventing regular bouts of hypoglycemia is frequent glucose monitoring. In the past, this often meant an inconvenient, painful procedure that involved pricking the fingertips to take a blood sample.

But recent technological breakthroughs have made glucose monitors much easier and more convenient to use. "A variety of features are available to accommodate patients' needs, such as very small meters for ease in carrying, preloaded strips to reduce the amount of dexterity needed to use the meter, alternate-site testing to avoid using the fingertips for the blood sample, large visual displays, and even audio readouts for patients with vision impairment," says Beverly Caskey, RPh, a Medco pharmacist who specializes in diabetes care.

Some patients with type 1 diabetes need almost constant glucose monitoring. And according to Gabriel I. Uwaifo, MD, associate professor of endocrinology in the department of medicine at the University of Mississippi in Jackson, advancements in the area of continuous glucose monitoring systems, or CGMS, have significantly helped their cause. "Continuous glucose monitoring systems are presently available for use in research settings and are being developed as partner systems for use with certain insulin pumps," he says. "This technology may eventually become part of standard care, particularly for brittle type 1 diabetics who often have frequent and severe hypoglycemic episodes."

well as make sure a spouse or significant other is trained in how to administer it. "If the hypoglycemia or the person's unresponsiveness persists even after the glucagon injection, seek emergency medical care," says Dr. Uwaifo.

■ **ASSESS THE CAUSE.** Once the episode ends, your work isn't quite done. Immediately determine why it happened and how to avoid a repeat, suggests Dr. Uwaifo. By carefully reviewing the factors right afterward, it should be pretty clear whether the cause was timing or amounts of medication or food, exercise, alcohol, or something else. "Furthermore, if the next meal is more than an hour away and the person had just consumed a significant amount of alcohol or completed a course of fairly vigorous exercise, he or she should take a small mixed meal or snack, such as a peanut butter and jelly sandwich with a glass of low-fat milk," says Dr. Uwaifo.

■ **KEEP TABS ON BLOOD SUGAR.** Because so many different factors can cause hypoglycemia and it's often unclear which one is at play, Dr. Uwaifo says that it's important to check your blood sugar frequently. This will give you a sense of how different activities affect your blood sugar and how you can adjust your activities accordingly. Also, says Caskey, "people with diabetes who have had recent hypoglycemic episodes should test their blood sugar before driving or exercising. Usually the level should be 100 mg/dL or greater before starting either of these activities."

■ **HAVE SNACKS AT THE READY.** If hypoglycemia hits, you don't want to be caught empty-handed. Caskey recommends having a readily available supply of sugar on hand, whether it's juice, soda, candy, sugar packets, or glucose tablets. Store them in your car, purse, briefcase, desk, and nightstand, she suggests.

■ **TIME IT RIGHT.** Most cases of diabetes-related hypoglycemia come down to poor timing, whether it's when you take your medication, when you eat, or when you exercise, says Dr. Uwaifo. That's why one of the most critical prevention strategies is shoring up any of these timing gaps. Be sure to eat the right amount of food around the time you take your medication or before exercising. Frequently checking your blood sugar will also help you sort out any timing issues.

The Diabetes Lowdown

Most of the time, a hypoglycemic episode begins with easily recognizable symptoms such as fatigue, weakness, dizziness, or confusion. But a handful of those who experience hypoglycemia have what is known as hypoglycemia unawareness, a state in which low blood sugar occurs without the warning signs. This can be quite dangerous, as the hypoglycemia often won't be evident until blood sugar is very low (less than 50 mg/dL, or milligrams per deciliter) and symptoms are so severe that the person can't self-administer carbohydrates. "If this happens while a person is asleep, driving, or operating other precision machinery, the consequences can be severe," says Gabriel I. Uwaifo, MD, associate professor of endocrinology in the department of medicine at the University of Mississippi in Jackson.

If you have hypoglycemia unawareness, you'll want to work with your doctor to deal with it safely, says Dr. Uwaifo. You may require more frequent checks of blood sugar, including before sleeping, driving, or operating machinery. In addition, you'll need to be even more vigilant about eating, exercising, and taking your medicine at the right times to prevent dangerous drops in blood sugar.

■ **GET BY WITH A LITTLE HELP FROM YOUR FRIENDS.** Hypoglycemia can render you powerless to help yourself in a frighteningly short amount of time. That's why it's critical to let loved ones, co-workers, or exercise buddies know about your diabetes and how to react if hypoglycemia occurs. This can be as simple as telling them where your emergency snacks are stashed or as involved as having them join you on a doctor's visit for instruction on giving glucagon injections.

■ **MAKE OTHERS AWARE.** Of course, you can't expect to have someone with you every waking hour. "That's why it's so important to wear a MedicAlert bracelet or wristband that identifies the wearer as diabetic and mentions the potential risk of hypoglycemia," says Dr. Uwaifo.

■ **STICK TO A SOUND DIET.** Ultimately, a sound diet presents the best way to balance blood sugar levels. According to Karen Miller-Kovach, RD, chief scientific officer at Weight Watchers International in Jericho, New York, this includes nonstarchy vegetables, whole grains and beans for fiber, and lean sources of protein. "The goal is to avoid a roller-coaster situation where hypoglycemia is treated with a large amount of simple sugars and spikes, then dives, and then repeats itself over and over," she says. "The best thing to do is to take the smallest amount needed to get through the episode, and then get back on a consistent eating pattern as soon as possible."

Diabetic Neuropathy

RIGHT NOW, as you read this, the muscles in your brain that cause your eyes to glide across the page are being jolted into action by more than a million tiny optic nerve fibers. Sailing on electrical current, these fibers relay visual information about the page—the black letters, the white background—from your retina to your brain's central cortex. The brain, in turn, responds to these signals by delivering messages to nerves that tell your body when to close your eyes, make them blink, jump to the next paragraph, and turn the page.

That's just a quick glimpse into the human nervous system, the most complex communication infrastructure in the world. This system is more complicated than any supercomputer you've ever heard of and faster than the quickest Internet modem money can buy.

Nerves relay information throughout the body within nanoseconds: They're responsible for mediating pain, stimulating muscles into action, and triggering organ function that modulates breathing, sweating, blood flow, heart rate, digestion, and other bodily functions. Without the proper interplay of nerves, various systems—such as the body's respiratory, circulatory, or digestive systems—fail to operate properly.

Chronic conditions like diabetes have the ability to damage the nervous system. When this happens, there is potential for serious problems throughout your body, from the top of your head to the tips of your toes.

What's the Connection?

Nerve damage, or neuropathy, can have many causes. Certain drugs prescribed for cancer, HIV/AIDS, Crohn's disease, and rheumatoid arthritis can inhibit nerve function. Viral infections, vitamin deficiencies, or physical injury also may cause nerve damage. A family history of neuropathy could increase your risk. However, if you have diabetes, nerve damage is likely due to two major factors: hyperglycemia and poor circulation. These factors contribute to a deteriorating loss of nerve function, which eventually leads to apoptosis, or nerve cell death.

When high levels of blood sugar attach to proteins and other molecules inside a nerve, the nerve's ability to metabolize sugar is compromised. Excess blood sugar also may contribute to clogged arteries that lead to poor circulation. When nerves cannot adequately metabolize sugar or get the nutrients they need from blood, their inner pathways and protective myelin coverings begin to break down.

The nerves that are most affected by diabetes-related neuropathy are the peripheral nerves, so called because they include all the nerves that extend from the central nervous system (the brain and spinal cord) into the body's limbs. Symptoms usually start in the sensory nerves, which distinguish touch and temperature, then may progress to the motor nerves (involving muscles) and, finally, the autonomic nerves (involving the internal organs), as explained below.

How Common Is It?

The longer you've had diabetes, the greater your chances for neuropathy. Statistics vary, but the consensus among physicians is that after 25 years, more than 50 percent of diabetes patients have the condition, with about half of them having autonomic neuropathy.

Patients with diabetes are also up to 30 times more likely to experience nerve compressions—swollen, irritated nerves within the nerve channel or tunnel that can exacerbate neuropathic pain—according to Gedge Rosson, MD, FACS, assistant professor of plastic surgery in the Division of Plastic, Reconstructive, and Maxillofacial Surgery at Johns Hopkins School of Medicine. You may experience the painful, debilitating effects of carpal or cubital tunnel syndrome in the wrist or funny bone, tarsal tunnel syndrome in the ankle, or fibular tunnel syndrome in the leg.

"Feelings of numbness, tingling, heaviness, or buzzing sensations in your outer extremities may indicate nerve compressions," Dr. Rosson says. "These symptoms often mimic traditional neuropathy, so it's wise to see a physician if you're feeling any discomfort."

What Is My Risk?

Neuropathy can have a significant impact on your quality of life. If you have pain or numbness in your feet or heaviness in your legs, you'll be less active and more likely to sit around on the couch all day. This poses a threat to your overall health, putting you at risk for countless other complications of diabetes.

To head off problems before they start, consult the list below. If you have one or more risk factors for neuropathy—besides diabetes or prediabetes—visit a physician for a full neurological evaluation.

- Poorly controlled blood sugar levels

- Male gender

- Overweight or obesity

- Nicotine use or alcohol abuse

- High carbohydrate consumption

- Vitamin B_{12} or folate deficiency

- Family history of nervous system disorders

- Autoimmune disease such as multiple sclerosis or rheumatoid arthritis

During your checkup, a physician or nerve specialist called a neurologist will evaluate your nerve function. You may be asked to undergo the following tests.

■ **FOOT EXAMINATION:** Feet are checked for pain, numbness, structural deformities, or slow-healing wounds that could cause infection. A health care provider may measure your response to pressure or vibration by tapping your foot with a tuning fork or other medical device (see Foot Complications on page 105).

■ **NERVE CONDUCTION STUDY:** Electrodes are placed on the skin to shock nerves with small electrical charges. Nerve impulses that appear slower or weaker than others may indicate damaged nerves.

■ **ELECTROMYOGRAPHY (EMG):** Usually performed in conjunction with nerve conduction, this test allows electrical currents to be seen on a computer monitor.

■ **QUANTITATIVE SENSORY TESTING (QST):** Nerve response to stimulus, such as pressure or vibration, is measured in problem areas that may exhibit pain, numbness, or abnormal sensations such as tingling.

■ **ULTRASOUND:** High-frequency sound waves produce a picture of the inside of the body and may reveal poor function of the heart, bladder, stomach, intestines, or other organs. If neuropathy is affecting internal organ function, you may be referred to a specialist.

What Should I Watch For?

The first signs of diabetic neuropathy usually show up in the longest peripheral nerves—those that are rooted in your spine and run down your leg to your toes. As a result, symptoms of nerve damage usually begin in the toes, the limbs farthest from the heart—and usually the hardest hit by poor circulation. The path of peripheral nerve damage follows a so-called stocking-and-glove pattern, beginning at the tips of the toes and fingers, then running up the legs and arms as the condition progresses.

Sensory nerves are usually the first to be affected. Some are large in diameter and conduct electricity faster than other nerves, so they may be most susceptible to metabolic changes or poor blood flow. Sensory nerves elicit feelings of pain to alert your body when an injury has occurred, so if they're damaged, you may lose the ability to detect pain or differentiate between hot and cold. Damaged nerves may cause abnormal sensations that patients describe as "burning, shooting aches," "pins and needles," "tingling," "ice cold," or "like bugs are crawling on the skin," as well as numbness. Symptoms are usually worse at night.

Motor nerves are affected next. These nerves help stimulate muscles that cause you to move your hands and feet or lift your arms and legs. Muscles that aren't properly stimulated by motor nerves will stop functioning well, and your legs may feel weak, tired, or heavy. If you then become less active, the muscle tissues will break down and atrophy, or waste away. That can lead to foot deformities, balance problems, and walking difficulties, such as an uncoordinated gait (as though you drank too much) called ataxia.

As neuropathy progresses throughout the peripheral nervous system, the autonomic nerves come into play. When these nerves are affected, organs fail to work properly, and you may experience the following symptoms.

- Vomiting or nausea

- Diarrhea, constipation, or bloating

- Problems urinating, or sensing when to "go"

- Shortness of breath, dizziness, or fainting

- Difficulty swallowing

- Dry, cracked hands or feet

- Swollen ankles or feet

- Excessive sweating

- Trouble seeing in the dark; sensitivity to light

- Sexual problems, including erectile dysfunction in men and vaginal dryness or lack of orgasm in women

- Inability to sense warning signs of hypoglycemia (fatigue, hunger, rapid heartbeat, or cold sweats), also known as hypoglycemia unawareness

- Depression

All three types of peripheral nerve damage can be very serious and even life threatening. A person who can't feel a cut on his or her foot risks infection that could spread to other parts of the body or lead to amputation. Someone unable to feel chest pains, limb paralysis, or other vital warning signs of a heart attack will not seek timely medical treatment.

What Can I Do about It?

"Maintaining tight glucose control is one of the best ways to prevent the progression of neuropathy," says Max J. Hilz, MD, FAAN, PhD, professor of neurology, medicine, and psychiatry at New York University School of Medicine and chair of the American Academy of Neurology's autonomic nerve section.

Consider the findings of the landmark Diabetes Control and Complications Trial of the 1990s. This study of 1,441 people with diabetes found that diabetic neuropathy could be prevented with intensive insulin therapy. The patients who took insulin at least three times a day—as opposed to once or twice daily—reduced their risk of developing neuropathy by 64 percent. They were also less likely to develop neuropathy than those who did not manage their diabetes with intensive insulin therapy.

Keeping blood sugar levels within normal ranges (or as directed by your physician) will help prevent complications of diabetes that cause nerve damage. If you begin an intensive insulin regimen, you might find that any neuropathy symptoms you're already experiencing become worse before they get better. This is normal and should subside once your body adjusts to the higher dosage, so don't give up. Controlling your blood sugar levels may not only help prevent the progression of neuropathy but might even reverse the effects. "Nerves that are damaged but not yet dead may be repaired through tight glucose control and a healthy lifestyle," Dr. Hilz says.

If you've had neuropathy for years, however, diabetes-controlling behavior is less likely to reverse the damage of neuropathy, but it will prevent your symptoms from getting worse. Damaged nerves that cause aching, tingling, or other abnormal sensations can be rehabilitated, but those that cause numbness have died and can never be repaired.

Listen to Your Endocrinologist

The best way to help preserve your nerves: Follow a healthy lifestyle. The Diabetes Prevention Program Study—which concluded in 2002 that improved diet and exercise habits sharply reduce the incidence of type 2 diabetes in people with impaired glucose tolerance—revealed a close association between fitness and organ function. The researchers also reported that getting more exercise reduces the risks of developing diabetes and related autonomic neuropathy. A 2006 Italian study echoed these findings, concluding that long-term exercise, such as daily walking on a treadmill at a brisk pace for at least 4 hours a week, helps prevent diabetic neuropathy.

If you have neuropathy in your feet, your balance may be compromised. So stick to low-impact activities such as swimming, bicycling, and rowing and avoid those that force you to make any sudden, abrupt movements that can cause injury—step aerobics, running, and kickboxing, to name a few.

If you're a smoker, here's another reason to quit: Smoking inhibits circulation throughout the body and may also adversely affect electrical charges between nerves. Excessive alcohol consumption inhibits nerve function, too.

Ease the Pain

Sometimes controlling your blood glucose and making necessary lifestyle changes aren't enough to ease extremely painful or irritating symptoms of neuropathy. Your physician may then recommend medications—but they don't replace healthy habits. "Patients want to hear that there's a magic bullet, a drug that's going to save them from the pain of neuropathy," Dr. Hilz says. "That just doesn't exist. Some pain medications are very effective but won't work well if you smoke, have high glucose levels, are overweight, or eat heavily processed, high-calorie foods."

With that in mind, review the treatments listed below. While there's currently no drug approved by the FDA to halt the progression of nerve damage, these strategies may ease pain or discomfort.

■ **NONNARCOTIC PAINKILLERS:** Taking daily aspirin, acetaminophen, or nonsteroidal anti-inflammatory drugs (NSAIDs) such as ibuprofen may reduce pain. Before using any of these drugs on a regular basis, consult your physician; for example, if you have kidney disease, you may need to avoid NSAIDs.

■ **TRICYCLIC ANTIDEPRESSANTS:** Studies show that some brain chemicals involved in depression, such as serotonin and norepinephrine, may also mediate pain. Antidepressants have been used off-label for years to treat neuropathy, and now some such as Cymbalta are newly FDA-approved for this use—so long as you don't have certain conditions such as vascular disease, hypotension, or angle-closure glaucoma.

■ **ANTISEIZURE MEDICATIONS:** Overactive, erratic nerves in the central nervous system cause seizures, and it's believed that the same phenomenon causes neuropathic pain in the peripheral nervous system. Thus, antiseizure drugs may tame erratic nerve signals and treat nerve damage. Those currently FDA-approved for neuropathy include Neurontin and Lyrica.

■ **TOPICAL CREAMS AND PATCHES:** Over-the-counter (OTC) products such as Ben-Gay that contain the active ingredient capsaicin—a chemical derived from chile peppers—have been found to significantly alleviate pain by blocking erratic nerve signals. Topical anesthetics such as the Lidoderm patch provide a continuous release of lidocaine, a numbing agent formerly reserved for use in doctor's offices, and may also bring relief.

Some painkilling remedies routinely performed in your doctor's office may also help. For example, biofeedback trains you to sense your body's own pain signals so that you can carry out appropriate treatment, and transcutaneous electrical nerve stimulation (TENS) uses small electrodes to shock nerves and block pain signals.

Surgical Relief

If you're diagnosed with nerve compression, surgery may not only alleviate those symptoms but also help with neuropathic pain. In fact, for up to 80 percent of people with neuropathy who undergo nerve decompression surgery, not only do symptoms resolve but some sensory feelings, such as touch and temperature sensitivity, are reclaimed.

This procedure is a relatively new option for diabetes patients with nerve damage. Dr. A. Lee Dellon, MD, PhD, of the Dellon Institutes for Peripheral Nerve Surgery, popularized this treatment in the 1990s after hand surgeons (and many of his own patients with both diabetes and nerve compressions) began reporting a decrease of neuropathic symptoms after routine carpal tunnel–release surgery. "Dr. Dellon decided to apply the same principles of tunnel release to various nerves throughout the body," says Dr. Rosson, who learned of the technique while completing a peripheral nerve surgery fellowship at the Dellon Institute in Baltimore.

During surgery, the roof of an affected nerve tunnel is cut away, giving the swollen nerve room to "breathe" and expand beyond its former covering. If the nerve presses on another nerve or sensitive area, it may be surgically moved to another location. Once the nerve is no longer constricted, swelling may cease and nerve function improves.

Beyond Pills and Procedures

Because pain is so subjective and varied, no two people experience the exact same symptoms. So when it comes to pain relief, what works well for your neighbor might not work well for you.

That's why it's important to try different treatment options, says Mark Allen Young, MD, FACP, director of the Oasis Center for Natural Pain Management in Baltimore, a licensed acupuncturist, and chairman of the department of physical medicine and rehabilitation at the Maryland Rehabilitation Center. "Some people find relief through traditional drug therapy and glucose control," he says. "Others find that herbal supplements or alternative treatments, such as acupuncture, acupressure, magnet therapy, massage, and meditation, and various types of movement—like yoga or tai chi—add greater therapeutic benefit to treatments."

Dr. Young urges people with diabetes to try traditional, nondrug remedies before moving on to pain medications and surgical measures for pain relief. The chart below lists several of the available remedies; some may work for you, while others won't. Before introducing any of these treatments into your pain management plan, be sure to consult your physician.

HERB/NUTRIENT	WHAT IT DOES	WHERE TO GET IT	INDICATIONS
Arnica montana	Eases muscle aches	Arnica flower tea, topical cream	Consult physician
Bromelain	Anti-inflammatory agent; aids turmeric and vitamin B6 (see below)	Pineapple/pineapple juice	1 glass (12 oz) 3 times a day (preferred method); 1 capsule (40 mg) 2 or 3 times a day
Cayenne (Capsicum annuum or frutescens)	Pain reliever	Red pepper	Topical cream applied several times a day (takes effect in 3–7 days); 1 capsule (30–120 mg) 3 times a day
Chamomile (Chamaemilum nobile/Matricaria recutita)	Mediates pain by affecting levels of serotonin and norepinephrine; fights inflammation; alleviates stress, tension	Chamomile tea	3 cups a day, each prepared with 2 tea bags in 1 cup boiling water (let steep 10 minutes)
Chromium	Helps insulin maintain blood glucose levels	Legumes, soybeans, lima beans, pinto beans, miso, tofu, cooked greens, mushrooms, pumpkin seeds, red meat, fish	1 capsule (minimum 25 mcg) a day
Copper	Reduces pain and inflammation; fights free radicals	Oysters, shellfish, liver, nuts, fruit, kidney, legumes, seeds, cereal, potatoes	Incorporate copper-rich foods into a balanced eating plan
Epigallocatechin gallate (EGCG)	Anti-inflammatory agent; relieves nerve pain	Green tea, green tea extract	3–4 cups tea a day (preferred method)

HERB/NUTRIENT	WHAT IT DOES	WHERE TO GET IT	INDICATIONS
Gamma-linolenic acid (GLA) (from omega-6 fatty acid family)	Relieves pain	Black currant seed oil, borage oil, evening primrose oil	1 capsule (100–150 mg) 3 times a day
Ginger (Zingiber officinale)	Enhances anti-inflammatory effects of bromelain	Gingerroot, ginger tea	100–300 mg a day
Lipoic acid	Aids nerve function in digestive tract and heart	Supplement	1 capsule (300–600 mg) a day
Omega-3 fatty acids (linolenic acids)	Assists nerve cell function; contains anti-inflammatory properties	Coldwater fish (tuna, salmon, flounder, halibut, striped bass), walnuts, wheat germ, wild game, flaxseed oil, grapeseed oil	Fish eaten at least 3 times a week; flaxseed oil, 1 tablespoon per day; grapeseed oil, follow label instructions (do not use if on blood thinners)
Passionflower (Passiflora incarnata)	Helps improve sleeping patterns; soothes nighttime symptoms of sensory neuropathy	Passionflower tea	2 cups tea a day (consult physician if taking sedatives)
Turmeric/curcumin (Curcuma longa)	May reduce inflammation associated with nerve compressions	Indian spices	1 capsule (400–600 mg) a day; regularly use spices with at least 95% curcumin (avoid turmeric/curcumin if you have gallstones, blood clots, or fertility problems)

HERB/NUTRIENT	WHAT IT DOES	WHERE TO GET IT	INDICATIONS
Vitamins B1 (thiamin) and B2 (riboflavin)	Improves nerve cell function; B2 aids efficacy of B6	Lean meat, leafy green vegetables such as spinach, whole grains, legumes, low-fat dairy products, acorn squash, watermelon, sunflower seeds	1 B1 capsule (1.4–50 mg) a day; 1 B2 capsule (1.1 mg) a day
Vitamin B5 (pantothenic acid)	Aids neurotransmitters; helps with glucose control	Whole grains, nuts, beans	Incorporate foods into a balanced eating plan
Vitamin B6 (pyridoxine)	Reduces muscle spasms, cramps, and inflammation; aids serotonin production	Meat, fish, milk, eggs, whole grains, vegetables, yeast, bananas, nuts, potatoes	1 capsule (2–100 mg) a day
Vitamin B12 (cobalamin)	Helps maintain nervous system; protects myelin nerve coating	Meat, liver, eggs, low-fat dairy products, leafy green vegetables, sea vegetables (seaweed), oysters, clams	1 capsule (1.5 mg) a day
Vitamin E (alpha-tocopherol)	Antioxidant/pain reliever	Avocado, wheat germ, safflower oil, leafy green vegetables, peanuts, nuts, soybeans, seeds, whole grains	1 capsule (15–1,000 mg) a day
Vitamin H (biotin)	Reduces muscle aches	Nuts, fruit, beef liver, milk, cauliflower, egg yolks, kidney, brewer's yeast	Incorporate foods into a balanced eating plan

Self-Care for Side Effects

If your neuropathy is the more progressive form that affects autonomic nerves, you may be wrestling with uncomfortable—and often embarrassing—symptoms, such as incontinence. Seeing a specialist and undergoing targeted treatment for your condition is crucial, but you may be able to alleviate some of your symptoms by practicing self-care strategies at home. The tips below may help with some of the most common side effects of autonomic neuropathy.

■ **BLADDER CONTROL:** Incontinence occurs when nerves that trigger urination stop functioning. You may not be able to sense when your bladder is full or have problems contracting your sphincter, which both allows urine to exit the body and prevents it from involuntarily escaping. Emptying your bladder every 2 to 3 hours—whether or not you sense the urge to go—can help prevent accidents. For more information, see Urinary Incontinence on page 76.

■ **GASTROINTESTINAL (GI) DYSFUNCTION:** Damaged nerves in the esophagus, stomach, intestines, or colon stop stimulating muscles to move food and waste down the GI tract. If this happens, you may suffer from nausea or vomiting. To alleviate these problems, eat four to six small meals a day, choosing foods that are low in fat and fiber. On the other hand, if you are constipated, increase your fiber intake. Be sure to consult your doctor before using any laxatives or antidiarrheal medications.

■ **LOW BLOOD PRESSURE:** If you feel lightheaded or dizzy when standing up or changing positions, you may have orthostatic hypotension—low blood pressure. This occurs when nerves that regulate blood pressure and heart rate work more slowly than normal. Blood may pool in your ankles, or you may experience difficulty catching your breath. To alleviate symptoms, rise slowly after sitting or lying; before you stand up, wiggle your toes and feet to get blood flowing to that area. Elastic stockings may also help with circulation problems. When sleeping at night, rest your head at a 30-degree angle.

■ **VISION PROBLEMS:** If your eyes have trouble adjusting to light when you walk into a dimly lit room, you may have focal neuropathy. This happens when autonomic nerves that dilate your pupil are damaged, so it takes longer for the pupil to widen and let light into the retina. For better vision, turn on lights when entering dark rooms, and use night-lights in hallways and bathrooms. For more information, see Vision Problems on page 37.

■ **DRY, CRACKED SKIN:** Sweat glands that stop functioning and adding moisture to your skin will cause your hands and feet to become painfully dry. Dry skin that splits open can become a pathway for infection, so keep your feet moisturized. For more information, see Foot Complications on page 117.

■ **HYPOGLYCEMIA UNAWARENESS:** If you've had diabetes for years and your autonomic nerves are damaged, normal signs of hypoglycemia—heart palpitations, cold sweats, anxiety, or tingling around your mouth—may fail to occur. To prevent a hypoglycemic event, check your blood sugar often, wear a diabetes ID bracelet, teach family members how to recognize and treat hypoglycemia, and always travel with a glucagon kit. For more information, see Hypoglycemia on page 116.

Polycystic Ovary Syndrome

SOME PREMENOPAUSAL WOMEN may think that a few missed periods a year is no big deal. And facial hair? Fixed with a trip to the salon. But when those two symptoms occur at the same time—especially when accompanied by obesity, too—they point to a serious medical condition: polycystic ovary syndrome.

One in 10 American women has PCOS, and many don't even know they have it. That's because doctors don't always recognize it, and taking birth control pills can mask the symptoms.

But PCOS isn't something to ignore. Not only does it cause infertility, it greatly increases a woman's risk of developing type 2 diabetes. When it goes untreated, PCOS also raises her risk for cancer.

The most common symptom is irregular menstruation. At least 80 percent of women with PCOS menstruate no more than eight times a year. The missed periods are a result of eggs failing to reach maturity; and because cysts cover the follicles of their ovaries, women with PCOS don't ovulate. For this reason, PCOS is the leading cause of infertility.

Without ovulation, women don't produce the hormone progesterone, which triggers the uterine lining to shed. Instead, the lining thickens, and this may lead to irregular, heavy bleeding and potentially to uterine cancer.

No wonder, then, that it's key that women learn to manage PCOS ASAP. It'll go a long way toward lowering risk of type 2 diabetes and other complications.

What's the Connection?

Doctors don't know exactly what causes PCOS, but there appears to be a strong genetic association: If a mother has it, her daughters also tend to have it, says Marcelle Cedars, MD, director of the University of California at San Francisco Center for Reproductive Health. Environmental factors, such as diet and weight gain, seem to play a role as well.

Doctors don't believe PCOS itself causes diabetes, but it creates risk factors that can lead to diabetes, Dr. Cedars says—notably, insulin resistance. If you have PCOS, you are more likely than other women to have insulin resistance. In fact, 30 to 70 percent of women with PCOS are thought to be less sensitive to insulin, Dr. Cedars says. And when that happens, you're more likely to gain weight—and you're 5 to 10 times more likely to develop type 2 diabetes.

Under normal circumstances, your pancreas produces insulin after you eat to usher glucose from your bloodstream to your muscles and tissues for energy. But when you're insulin resistant, your body doesn't respond to a normal amount of the hormone, and your pancreas churns out much more in an attempt to keep blood sugar levels normal. Elevated insulin levels drive fat deposits to the abdomen and further increase insulin levels. When your body is no longer able to maintain normal blood sugar levels, you develop type 2 diabetes.

Insulin also seems to be the culprit for hirsutism—unwanted hair growth in women. Insulin works with luteinizing hormone in your body to enhance the production of androgens. The high levels of these male hormones cause hair to grow where you'd rather it didn't (face, torso, back, upper arms and legs, or lower abdomen), acne, and male-pattern baldness. Insulin also prevents testosterone from binding with sex hormone–binding globulin, leaving a higher amount of free testosterone hanging around in a woman's system.

Being insulin resistant over a long period of time also raises your risk of heart disease. Women who have PCOS are more likely to have high blood pressure, high cholesterol, liver disease, sleep apnea, and cardiovascular problems.

How Common Is It?

Experts say that women with PCOS represent the largest group of women at risk for diabetes and heart disease. In one study, 21 percent of 38 women with diabetes had PCOS. Another study evaluated 30 women with type 2 diabetes and found that 27 percent, or one in four, had PCOS, significantly higher than what's seen in women without diabetes.

In the Nurses' Health Study of 116,000 women ages 25 to 42, women who had irregular menstrual periods (but weren't necessarily diagnosed with PCOS) were about 2½ times more likely to have type 2 diabetes, compared with women who had regular periods.

What Is My Risk?

To assess your risk of PCOS, consider these questions.

1. Do you have eight or fewer menstrual periods a year?

2. Do you have facial hair and acne?

3. Are you obese, or is your waist circumference more than 35 inches?

■ **YOU ANSWERED YES TO ALL THREE:** Although there are other signs of PCOS, these are the major symptoms doctors focus on. Your doctor can confirm the diagnosis by testing your hormone levels and performing other tests.

■ **YOU ANSWERED YES TO LESS THAN THREE:** Doctors tend to look for all three symptoms when they're evaluating a woman for PCOS. But if you have irregular menstrual periods, you should consult your doctor. "Irregular menstrual periods are a vital sign for an endocrine problem," says Kathleen Hoeger, MD, associate professor of obstetrics and gynecology at the University of Rochester Medical Center in New York. Facial hair is another red flag to discuss with your doctor.

When to See the Doctor

Whatever your age, it's important to see your gynecologist or an endocrine specialist if you have irregular periods and signs of hirsutism.

Many women discover they have PCOS soon after puberty. Although it's common for girls to experience irregular menstrual periods for the first year or two after menstruation starts, if it continues beyond 3 years, it may point to a problem. Another red flag is facial hair with the onset of puberty. "These things should trigger a doctor's visit," says Kathleen Hoeger, MD, associate professor of obstetrics and gynecology at the University of Rochester Medical Center in New York.

But it's possible for your doctor to miss PCOS, especially if you're on birth control pills to regulate your periods. In one study, researchers discovered that 25 percent of the women who had PCOS were undiagnosed, even though they were patients at a clinic that specialized in the syndrome.

To diagnose this condition, your doctor may perform a pelvic exam and order an ultrasound to check for cysts on your ovaries, as well as a blood test to measure testosterone (which tends to be elevated in PCOS), insulin, and glucose levels. Because women with PCOS also tend to have high cholesterol, your doctor may check those levels as well.

Once you've been diagnosed, you might be prescribed birth control pills to manage the symptoms of acne, hair growth, and irregular periods, plus insulin-sensitizing drugs if needed. If you're trying to conceive, you may need to take medications to improve ovulation, but losing as little as 10 percent of your overall weight can induce ovulation.

What Should I Watch For?

Signs and symptoms include eight or fewer menstrual periods a year; infertility; weight gain; acne; male pattern baldness; a waist measurement greater than 35 inches; dark skin patches in the folds of the neck, armpits, waistline, and groin; and hair on the face, torso, back, upper arms and legs, or lower abdomen.

Hirsutism occurs in 70 percent of PCOS cases, but what it looks like varies from woman to woman. Some women grow so much hair that they have to shave every day, says Dr. Hoeger. Others can take care of the problem with periodic trips to the salon for hair-removal treatments.

What Can I Do about It?

■ **SET A MODERATE WEIGHT LOSS GOAL.** Making lifestyle changes that will help you lose weight is the best prescription you can write for yourself. "Diet and exercise are part of the standard recommendation for PCOS," Dr. Cedars says.

Doctors suspect that for a woman who's genetically predisposed to PCOS, obesity could trigger the disease to take hold. At least 50 percent of women with PCOS are obese, which significantly increases the risk of insulin resistance and type 2 diabetes. Weight gain can also mess up the menstrual cycle.

Skeptical that losing weight will really help? Don't be. Up to 60 percent of women will start having regular periods when they lose weight, Dr. Cedars says.

Even a little weight loss will bring benefits. Studies have found that losing just 5 to 10 percent of your weight and keeping it off will help women ovulate, improve insulin sensitivity, decrease hair growth, and lower the risk of diabetes. Dr. Hoeger says that women in her clinic have experienced long-term results when they maintain a moderate weight loss.

Another reason to drop extra pounds: A 2005 study found that two out of three women with PCOS also have nonalcoholic fatty liver disease, which is caused by fat accumulating in the liver and is associated with obesity. Obese women with PCOS were at least two to three times more likely to have the disease, compared with lean, healthy women.

■ **BANISH BELLY FAT.** PCOS causes fat to settle around your middle, which puts you at higher risk of diabetes and heart disease—even if you're not overweight or obese. And visceral fat around your abdominal organs makes you more likely to be insulin resistant, Dr. Hoeger says. Experts suggest aiming for a waist circumference of 35 inches or less.

You doubtless know that what goes in your mouth affects what lands around your abs, but you might be surprised to learn it's not just about calories. Researchers conducting the Framingham Nutrition Studies found that women who chose the least nutritious food—even when they ate 400 fewer calories— had 2½ times higher risk of abdominal obesity than women who ate more calories but made healthier choices. The poorer eaters also were at higher risk of getting diabetes and suffering a heart attack.

■ **CURB SIMPLE SUGARS.** Ignore all those PCOS diet books that urge you to go low-carb; no studies suggest low-carbohydrate diets are better for women with PCOS, Dr. Hoeger says. She tells her patients to instead focus on a low-glycemic index diet to curb PCOS symptoms and control blood sugar levels. That means taking simple sugars off the menu but adding high-fiber complex carbohydrates. Swap foods made with white flour and refined sugar with fresh fruits, vegetables, whole grains, lean protein, and low-fat dairy products. Here's a sample PCOS-friendly food plan.

- Breakfast: whole grain cereal with fat-free milk *or* an egg with a whole wheat English muffin and trans-fat-free spread

- Lunch: tuna sandwich made with low-fat mayo on whole grain bread with raw veggies and low-fat dip *or* low-sodium soup with salad and a slice of whole grain bread

- Dinner: 3 ounces grilled salmon, chicken, or beef tenderloin with a baked potato or brown rice and steamed veggies

- Snacks: fruit, low-fat yogurt, popcorn, or graham crackers

■ **GET MOVING ALMOST EVERY DAY.** Aim to exercise for at least 30 minutes five or six days a week, Dr. Cedars says; ideally, choose a combination of aerobic and muscle-building moves. Pushing harder will pay off. A study published in the *Journal of Applied Physiology* revealed that increasing the intensity during short intervals throughout your workout can help you burn up to 36 percent more fat. If you bike or walk for an hour, increase your pace for 1 minute out of every 5 to burn a third more calories.

Building muscle will do more than shape you up and slim you down. Muscle mass utilizes insulin better than fat does, Dr. Cedars says.

■ **GET REGULAR DIABETES TESTS.** You should be screened for diabetes with a glucose tolerance test as soon as you're diagnosed with PCOS, whether that's age 16 or 35, Dr. Cedars says. If the results are normal, you should repeat the test every 3 to 5 years.

■ **KEEP CHOLESTEROL IN CHECK.** Many women with PCOS have low "good" HDL cholesterol and high triglycerides, and that puts them at higher risk for getting heart disease or suffering a stroke before age 60. Dr. Hoeger recommends getting your cholesterol checked when you're diagnosed with PCOS. If it's normal, get retested every 1 to 3 years.

■ **PROTECT YOURSELF FROM ENDOMETRIAL CANCER.** With PCOS, your ovaries are making estrogen all the time, which stimulates the endometrium, or the uterine lining, to grow. Normally, the lining is shed every month during menstruation, but when you have PCOS, you don't produce the hormone progesterone, which triggers the lining to shed, allowing your endometrium to overgrow. That puts you at higher risk for endometrial cancer. Your doctor can prescribe the hormone progestin to allow the lining to shed and protect against endometrial cancer, Dr. Cedars says.

Stroke

IN THE SIMPLEST OF TERMS, stroke is to the head and brain what a heart attack is to the chest and heart. Though each affects different areas, the mechanisms at work are essentially the same. And if you have diabetes, what increases your risk of heart disease and high blood pressure also tends to elevate your stroke risk.

What's the Connection?

When a stroke occurs, it generally happens in two distinct ways, says Daisy Merey, MD, PhD, author of *Don't Be a Slave to What You Crave* and *The Palm Beach Diet Doctor's Prescription*. "Stroke may occur when an artery in the brain bursts due to hypertension or because a clot forms in the brain that clogs up an artery and prevents blood flow," she says. "The area of the brain that did not receive blood—and therefore nutrients—dies; depending on which area of the brain is affected, different disabilities occur."

Diabetes can cause either scenario to play out. "High blood sugar damages blood vessels and increases the chance for blood clots to form," says Beverly Caskey, RPh, a Medco pharmacist who specializes in diabetes care. "Insulin resistance, a common part of type 2 diabetes, also increases the risk and rate of atherosclerosis, or hardening of the arteries. Many patients with diabetes also have high cholesterol, which can contribute to coronary artery disease, heart attack, and stroke."

The tangled web of connections between obesity, diabetes, heart disease, high blood pressure, and stroke can be a difficult mess to sort through. But what's most important to consider is that even though the causes are unclear, the strategies for preventing any of these interrelated maladies are clear and consistent. "Diabetes is a complex condition with many interrelated issues that make it difficult to discern what caused the actual damage," says Caskey. "What is known is that control of as many of the conditions as possible—blood pressure, cholesterol, maintaining a healthy weight, exercising, and eating nutritiously—helps to limit the risk of stroke."

How Common Is It?

Just like heart disease and high blood pressure, stroke is an ominous threat to a person with diabetes. "The risk of stroke is two to four times greater in people with diabetes, compared with the general population," says Caskey. "And more than 65 percent of deaths in diabetic patients are caused by heart disease or stroke."

In addition, people with diabetes often have far worse outcomes than those without the disease. "When someone has a stroke caused by a clogged artery, the oxygen supply to the brain is cut off," says Judith Stanton, MD, an instructor in the internal medicine residency program at Alameda County Medical Center in California. "Often the damage is limited because other arteries can usually deliver oxygen to the area. In people with diabetes, however, many of the surrounding arteries are also affected by atherosclerosis and impair blood flow to the brain." This combination of increased risk of stroke and poorer outcome creates a scary prospect for many people with diabetes.

What Is My Risk?

Since the causes of stroke are nearly identical to those of heart disease, it stands to reason that the risk factors are also quite similar, including family history, smoking, obesity, and inactivity. Stroke does present a few additional things to keep an eye on, however.

You should be aware of a personal or family history of blood clots because many strokes are caused by clotting in the blood vessels of the brain. Also, alert your doctor if you feel any type of pain or discomfort in your legs when walking. When the pain is circulation related, it is known as intermittent claudication and is caused by peripheral arterial disease, a condition in which narrowed arteries reduce blood flow to the limbs. PAD is a classic warning sign for stroke. (For more information on PAD, see page 106.)

The yes-or-no questions below will give you a sense of your risk of stroke and what you may want to discuss with your doctor. The more questions to which you answer yes, the greater your risk.

- Do you have a family history of stroke or heart disease?

- Do you smoke?

- Do you have high blood pressure?

- Is your total cholesterol greater than 200 mg/dL (milligrams per deciliter)?

- Is your A1C (blood sugar level) above 7 percent?

- Is your BMI (body mass index) greater than 25?

- Is your waistline greater than 34 inches (if you're a woman) or 40 inches (if you're a man)?

- Would you describe yourself as inactive?

- Do you have heart disease?

- Have you ever had blood clots?

- Do you ever have pain in the leg muscles when walking?

- Are you over age 75?

What Should I Watch For?

Unfortunately, stroke shares another somewhat frightening similarity with both heart disease and high blood pressure. It is asymptomatic, which means it often exhibits no symptoms until a full-blown stroke occurs. "Like many of the other complications of diabetes, stroke is often silent," says Dr. Stanton. "It is therefore extremely important to be assessed for risk factors—hypertension, kidney disease, high cholesterol, and others—and treated even if you don't have any symptoms."

Even so, sometimes stroke will give you warning signs immediately before it strikes. If you (or a loved one) experience any of the symptoms mentioned

When to See the Doctor

- If you experience some combination of numbness or tingling in the hands or feet, temporary numbness or weakness anywhere in the body, abnormal vision, slurred speech, abnormal gait, headache, muscle weakness, or lack of coordination, you could be having a stroke and should seek immediate medical attention.

- If you are overweight or inactive; smoke; have had blood clots; have leg pain; have a family history of heart disease or stroke; or have high cholesterol, blood pressure, or blood sugar, you should be under a doctor's close supervision for the risks associated with diabetes and stroke.

- If you have diabetes and are concerned about your stroke risk, ask your doctor about a routine blood test to check for high levels of blood coagulation factors.

below, seek immediate medical attention. Stroke is an emergency, and a few minutes can spell the difference between life and death.

- Numbness or tingling in the hands or feet (peripheral neuropathy)

- Temporary numbness or weakness anywhere in the body (including the face)

- Abnormal vision

- Slurred speech

- Abnormal gait

- Sudden severe headache

- Muscle weakness

- Lack of coordination

What Can I Do about It?

It's true that 65 percent of deaths in diabetic patients are due to heart attack or stroke, but it doesn't have to be that way. "Controlling blood pressure, blood sugar, and cholesterol; smoking cessation; exercise; and weight control will all help reduce one's risk of stroke," says Rani G. Whitfield, MD, a physician in private practice in Baton Rouge, Louisiana, and a spokesperson for the American Heart Association. Here are some specific ways to accomplish all that.

ASK YOUR DOCTOR ABOUT MEDICATION. Of all the factors in minimizing stroke risk, Dr. Whitfield says that the big two are undoubtedly blood pressure and cholesterol. Though the role of diet and exercise in achieving healthy numbers should not be overlooked, it's also important to realize the key role that medication can play. "Several recent landmark studies have shown that reducing blood pressure and cholesterol through medication decreases one's incidence of stroke," he says.

Among those studies is the HOPE (Heart Outcomes Prevention Evaluation) study, which showed that blood pressure control through medication reduced the incidence of death, heart attack, and stroke by 22 percent among almost 10,000 participants. A more recent UK study, the ASCOT study (Anglo-Scandinavian Cardiac Outcomes Trial), showed that the combination of a calcium-channel blocker and ACE inhibitor for blood pressure, along with a statin for cholesterol, cut the risk of heart attack and stroke in half among a group of 19,000 people.

■ **GET AN ESTIMATE.** The American Heart Association (AHA) recommends seeing your doctor as early as age 20 for heart disease risk-factor screening. This includes getting your blood pressure, BMI, waist circumference, and pulse checked every 2 years and your cholesterol and glucose checked every 5 years. The screening determines your risk estimate, which tells you your risk of developing heart disease within the next 10 years, or the next 5 years if you're over 40.

If you're particularly concerned about your stroke risk, ask your doctor to check your blood for coagulation factors. "If you have excess coagulation factors such as fibrinogen (a protein that supports blood coagulation), then you might be at increased risk of stroke," says Dr. Merey. Two other strangely named blood components, Von Willebrand factor and factor VIIIc, may raise stroke risk, as can a high white blood cell count. Your doctor can usually detect these through a routine blood test.

■ **TAKE AN ASPIRIN.** In addition to your other medication, taking a low-dose (75 to 150 milligrams) aspirin every day may help prevent the clots that cause strokes, says Dr. Merey. Just be sure to check with your doctor first.

■ **FOLLOW A DOUBLE-DUTY DIET.** The basics of a healthy diabetes diet are also the basics of a heart-healthy diet, says Wahida Karmally, RD, director of nutrition at the Irving Center for Clinical Research at Columbia-Presbyterian Medical Center in New York City and a member of the AHA's nutrition committee. And it's not complicated. "The easiest way to explain the perfect diabetic diet is to describe a plate," she says. "Half of it should be covered in brightly colored vegetables; a quarter of the plate, or about 3 ounces, should be lean meat; and the other quarter should be a source of whole grain, such as rice, bread, or pasta."

■ **HALT THE SALT.** The other component of the heart-healthy diet is to cut back on salt—way back. "A low-salt diet can lower blood pressure by 10 points," says Dr. Stanton. And lower blood pressure equals lower stroke risk.

■ **BANISH BOOZE AND STOP SMOKING.** Some studies have indicated a heart-protective, cholesterol-lowering benefit from moderate drinking. But exceed "moderate" by even a little, and that benefit quickly turns into a liability—for the heart and for the rest of the body. Many experts deem the risks too great to recommend imbibing at all. Stick to one drink a day if you're a woman, two if you're a man. As for smoking, it almost goes without saying that quitting is a must.

■ **EAT YOUR OMEGA-3S.** The omega-3 fatty acids EPA and DHA (eicosapentaenoic acid and docosahexaenoic acid)—which are found in fatty fish such as salmon, herring, and mackerel; fish oil supplements; and flaxseed—have

The Diabetes Lowdown

While everyone needs to take steps to reduce their risk of stroke, this is particularly vital for African Americans, says Rani G. Whitfield, MD, a physician in private practice in Baton Rouge, Louisiana, and a spokesperson for the American Heart Association. "More than 100,000 African Americans suffer from stroke each year," he says. "In addition, African Americans are two times more likely than white Americans to suffer from a stroke."

Higher rates of high blood pressure, diabetes, and sickle-cell anemia may be partially to blame for the raised risk. Dr. Whitfield advises African Americans concerned about their risk of stroke to consult a doctor about how best to protect themselves.

natural blood-thinning properties to prevent strokes caused by clots, says Dr. Merey. Strive for at least two servings of fatty fish a week or 1,000 to 2,000 milligrams of fish oil daily. As usual, talk to your doctor before starting any supplement.

■ **GET UP AND MOVING.** Last but very far from least, exercise is essential for minimizing stroke and other cardiovascular disease risks. "Exercise helps keep blood sugar regular, raises HDL, and lowers blood pressure," says Dr. Stanton. "We know regular aerobic exercise improves cardiovascular fitness and decreases risk of heart disease and stroke by decreasing atherosclerosis and improving circulation. Exercise also naturally aids weight loss or prevents weight gain, which in turn lowers blood pressure, helps improve glycemic control, lowers cholesterol, and decreases risk of heart disease. Central obesity [weight carried around your waistline] is a risk factor in itself for heart disease and stroke."

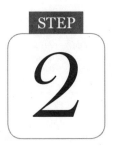

STEP

2

NAVIGATE THE DIABETES DANGER ZONES

Abdominal Fat

■ **WHAT'S WRONG:** I've got an apple shape.

■ **WHY IT MATTERS:** Carrying fat around your middle rather than in your hips is a risk factor for both diabetes and heart disease. In fact, researchers are starting to think that waist circumference may be one of the most important determinants of overall health.

■ **THE GOOD NEWS:** With a little extra effort, you can banish belly fat. In a 2005 study from Duke University, a group of exercisers shrank their belly fat by 7 percent just by walking at a higher intensity (an effort of between 6 and 8 on a scale of 1 to 10).

WE'VE ALWAYS BEEN TOLD that apples are good for our health—they keep the doctor away, provide heart-healthy fiber and vitamins, and clean our teeth when we can't grab a toothbrush. However, an apple is not such a good thing if it describes the shape you see in the mirror. The fat that parks itself on your abdomen, creating the apple shape, is more dangerous to your health—particularly for heart disease and diabetes risk—than the fat on your arms, hips, or butt. When it comes to storing fat, it pays to be a pear.

Why is belly fat so detrimental? For one thing, fat stored around the waist is more likely to affect lipids in the blood and clog up arteries than fat stored around the thighs and hips, says Ralph Felder, MD, PhD, section chief for cardiovascular nutrition, cardiology fellowship program at Banner Good Samaritan Medical

Center in Phoenix and author of the *Bonus Years Diet*. Plus, belly fat (known in the medical community as inter-abdominal fat or visceral adiposity) seems to increase insulin resistance and the risk of diabetes.

"The fat on your abdomen is different from the fat on other parts of your body in that it carries many more hormones, such as leptin, which helps propagate diabetes," says Eric Yan, MD, physician nutrition specialist at Valens Medical in Irvine, California. And abdominal fat contains lower levels of adiponectin, a protective hormone that lowers insulin resistance and inflammation; a lack of it further increases the risk for diabetes, he says.

In addition, abdominal fat is part of a constellation of modifiable risk factors called metabolic syndrome. Also known as the deadly quartet, metabolic syndrome consists of visceral adiposity—specifically, a waist greater than 35 inches in a woman and 40 inches in a man; high blood pressure (above 135/85 mm Hg, or millimeters of mercury); high cholesterol and triglycerides; and elevated blood sugar. "Metabolic syndrome is a prediabetic condition, so most people with visceral adiposity are prediabetic; and eventually, most people with visceral adiposity go into diabetes," says Fred Vagnini, MD, medical director of the Cardiovascular Wellness Centers of New York. "Metabolic syndrome is extra lethal because people with the condition are not only at risk for diabetes but also for heart attack, stroke, Alzheimer's disease, and many types of cancer."

Abdominal fat appears to be so detrimental to heart health and diabetes risk, in fact, that a recent study published in the *Lancet* revealed that the waist-to-hip ratio, or WHR (your waist measurement divided by your hip measurement), is three times more effective at predicting risk for cardiovascular disease than the body mass index (BMI), the ratio of weight to height that's commonly used to assess overall health. It is important to note that you can be at a healthy weight by BMI standards and look relatively thin, but if a significant portion of those pounds sits on your middle, you may still be at risk for a number of health conditions.

"Furthermore, if obesity is redefined using WHR instead of BMI, the proportion of 'abdominally obese' people at risk for heart attack increases by threefold, according to the *Lancet* researchers," Dr. Felder says.

It's not the belly fat directly under the skin that seems to be the problem—it's the fat that lies deep in the abdomen. "A paper published in the *New England Journal of Medicine* a few years ago looked at people who had a significant amount of subcutaneous fat removed from their abdominal walls through liposuction, and they really didn't show any improvement in health," says Barry J. Goldstein, MD, PhD, director of the division of endocrinology, diabetes, and metabolic diseases at Jefferson Medical College of Thomas Jefferson University in Philadelphia.

Deflating the Spare Tire

The best thing you can do to protect your heart and your risk for diabetes is to avoid putting on abdominal fat in the first place. "Once you've generated fat tissue, you can't destroy it—you can only shrink it," says Alan Marcus, MD, a physician in private practice in Laguna Hills, California, who specializes in diabetes management and endocrinology. But if you've already packed a few pounds around your middle, you'll still do yourself a world of good by taking off some of it.

And you don't have to lose much to make a difference in your health. "If you lose only 10 percent of your body weight, you can drastically reduce your risk for diabetes and other conditions," Dr. Vagnini says.

The tips below will help you lose weight throughout your entire body, including your abdomen. "Despite the claims that devices that shake or massage belly fat will shrink your middle, no one has really come up with one strategy per se that specifically targets abdominal fat over other types of fat," Dr. Goldstein says.

■ **ASSESS YOUR AB FAT.** To see where you stand in terms of abdominal fat, take a flexible tape measure and wrap it snugly (not tightly) around the widest part of your waist. Then measure the widest part of your hips. Compare the two numbers; if your waist is the same as or bigger than your hips, you're carrying too much weight on your stomach.

■ **IF YOU SMOKE, STOP.** Although smokers generally have lower BMIs than nonsmokers do, they have more abdominal fat. In a British study of 21,828 men and women published in the August 2005 issue of *Obesity Research,* the researchers discovered that current smokers had the largest waist-to-hip ratios, and those who had never smoked had the smallest. Among current and former smokers, the size of the ratio depended on the number of cigarettes smoked. Still smoking? Quit now for a head start on minimizing your middle.

■ **CREATE A BELLY-SHRINKING BALANCE.** If you have excess abdominal fat that puts you at risk for metabolic syndrome and diabetes, the American Diabetes Association suggests you eat a diet composed of about 25 percent protein, 45 percent carbohydrates, and 30 percent fat (primarily unsaturated).

■ **WHEN IT COMES TO DIETARY FAT, GO MONO.** Not all fats are created equal. Studies show that although monounsaturated fats serve up the same number of calories as other types of dietary fat, they're less likely to end up as extra pounds and abdominal fat. "Researchers compared the weight loss results from one group of people following a diet of large amounts of fish, olive oil, vegetables, and fruits with another group of people who were sticking to low-fat and high-carbohydrate diets," Dr. Felder explains. "They found that those following the fish/olive oil/vegetables and fruit diet shed excess pounds from both the upper and lower body, but the other group mainly lost fat from the lower body."

■ **MUNCH ON A MEDITERRANEAN DIET.** Monounsaturated fats are a big part of the Mediterranean diet, an eating plan that has also been shown to help shrink belly fat. When it comes to losing abdominal fat and overall weight, Dr. Vagnini recommends a modified low-carbohydrate Mediterranean diet of "fruits, vegetables, whole grains, low-fat protein, olive oil, and red wine." In addition to lowering the risk of diabetes, the Mediterranean diet has been shown to lower blood pressure and help prevent Alzheimer's disease and metabolic syndrome.

■ **SKIMP ON SIMPLE CARBS.** Dr. Vagnini recommends you avoid sweets and other simple sugars. "Get rid of the cookies, candies, doughnuts, ice cream, and cake (except maybe on your birthday), and reduce the bread, pasta, rice, potatoes, cereals, fruits, and fruit juices," he says. The degree of restriction depends on your weight and your blood sugar—the more you weigh and the higher your blood sugar, the more you need to steer clear of simple carbs.

■ **BE CHOOSY ABOUT VEGGIES.** Vegetables are generally great for weight loss because they deliver so much nutrition for relatively few calories. But they're not all created equal in terms of abdominal fat and diabetes risk, Dr. Vagnini says. You can eat broccoli, peppers, onions, cauliflower, celery, cucumbers, spinach, and so on pretty much without restraint. On the other hand, starchy vegetables—such as corn, beets, carrots, lima beans, potatoes, and sweet potatoes—tend to act more like carbohydrates in your body and so should be limited.

■ **MOVE IT TO LOSE IT.** Contrary to popular belief, it's not crunches that take most of the weight off your abdomen; it's cardiovascular exercise. Luckily, you don't have to move much to start lightening up. "Even if you just walk for 10 to 15 minutes after you eat, it's better than nothing," says Martha Funnell, RN, CDE, a clinical nurse specialist and codirector of the Behavioral, Clinical, and Health Systems Research Core at the University of Michigan Diabetes Research and Training Center.

If you haven't been active for a while, be sure to talk to your health care professional about exercise before you begin. Then start slowly, and increase your total time by 1 to 3 minutes each week, Funnell suggests. Ideally, build up to 30 minutes of moderate activity, such as brisk walking, 4 or 5 days a week. Other great cardio options: aerobics classes, dancing, tennis, racquetball, golf (if you walk the course), and jogging.

■ **STEP UP YOUR WORKOUT.** Although you'll no doubt lose weight with moderate exercise, to specifically target belly fat, you may want to push yourself a little harder. In an 8-month Duke University study of 175 overweight adults, a third of the participants exercised at a low intensity, another third worked out at a higher intensity, and the remaining third didn't exercise at all. At the end of the study, the nonexercisers gained 8.6 percent abdominal fat, and the low-intensity exercisers fended off additional abdominal pounds, despite gaining an average of 1.5 pounds. But the greatest intensity brought the greatest results: Those folks lost an average of 6 pounds *and* shrunk their belly fat by 7 percent.

■ **DON'T FORGET THE FOOD FACTOR.** Your workouts won't banish belly fat if you're still eating with abandon. "Exercise is important, but it cannot begin to take the place of diet changes," says Neal Barnard, MD, adjunct associate professor of medicine at George Washington University School of Medicine and Health Services and author of *Dr. Neal Barnard's Program for Reversing Diabetes*.

■ **FEAST ON FIBER.** Fiber acts like negative calories: Each 14 grams of fiber that you add to your diet per day cuts your total calorie intake by about 10 percent. High-fiber foods fill you up faster, so you stop eating sooner. Plus, fiber keeps you regular, so you're less likely to have a constipated, bloated belly.

One of the easiest ways to incorporate fiber into your diet is by choosing high-fiber breads. "Check the label—if the bread has at least 5 grams of fiber per slice, it's high in fiber," says Donna Rice, RN, CDE, a past president of the American Association of Diabetes Educators. Other fiber-packed foods include whole wheat pasta, brown rice, and cruciferous vegetables such as broccoli, Brussels sprouts, and cauliflower. Aim for at least 25 grams of fiber per day.

Dr. Felder suggests the following ways to sneak more fiber into your diet.

- Add whole grains to vegetables, soups, and stews. Slip some bulgur wheat into casseroles or stir-fries, and use barley in soups and stews.

- Make whole grain rice pilaf with a mixture of wild rice, barley, brown rice, broth, and spices. For even more fiber, stir in some nuts or dried fruit.

- Substitute whole wheat or oat flour for half of the flour in pancakes, muffins, waffles, and other flour-based recipes.

- Make meat loaf with whole grain bread or cracker crumbs.

- Use rolled oats or crushed unsweetened whole grain cereal as breading for baked chicken, fish, veal, or eggplant.

■ **BONE UP ON DAIRY.** In a study of 34 obese people, those who ate three servings of fat-free yogurt per day lost 22 percent more weight, 61 percent more body fat, and 81 percent more belly fat than people who ate the same amount of calories minus the dairy. Why? Dairy products seem to lower levels of cortisol, a stress hormone that causes you to store fat on your belly.

■ **SUCK DOWN SOME SEAWEED.** One possible reason Japanese people are so slim: A certain type of kelp called wakame, which is widely consumed in Japan, seems to shrink belly fat. Researchers found that fucoxanthin, the brown pigment in seaweed, helped mice and rats lose 5 to 10 percent of their weight by shrinking belly fat. Fucoxanthin appears to stimulate a protein found in abdominal fat that causes fat burning. Eating sushi wrapped in seaweed and other kelp-containing dishes may help shrivel your belly—and your risk for diabetes.

Dining Out

■ **WHAT'S WRONG:** I eat most of my meals away from home.

■ **WHY IT MATTERS:** A steady diet of restaurant food, especially fast food, tends to be full of fat and sodium and shy on fiber. The nutritional imbalance can mess with your blood sugar and pack on pounds—and typical extralarge portions compound the calories.

■ **THE GOOD NEWS:** Sticking with smaller portions can have big benefits for controlling weight and, therefore, diabetes risk.

FROM THE TIME WE WERE KIDS, whether it meant a ride on the Fry Guys merry-go-round at McDonald's or waiting in the backseat while a carhop on roller skates glided over with our meals on a tray, we've been taught that dining out is fun. And props or not, let's face it—it really *is* fun. You get a multitude of delectable choices, tasty drinks and wines, and friends or family and good conversation.

But the people part aside, dining out can be detrimental to your health, particularly if you have type 2 diabetes or are at risk for it. "When you eat out, you have no idea of the hidden oils, added carbohydrates, or quality of the nutrients you are eating, so you are behind the eight ball right away," says Francine Kaufman, MD, head of the Center for Diabetes, Endocrinology, and Metabolism at Childrens Hospital Los Angeles.

Plus, the portion sizes at restaurants are way out of control. "I went to a restaurant lately and saw a baked potato that was the size of some people's pets," says Alan Marcus, MD, a physician in private practice in Laguna Hills, California, who specializes in diabetes management and endocrinology. For example, the typical soda at a fast-food restaurant used to be 8 ounces; now a large soda is 32 ounces, a difference of 260 calories. A Double Quarter Pounder with Cheese, large fries, and a large chocolate shake—a typical meal for many Americans—add up to 2,080 calories and 90 grams of fat, more than most people need for the whole day. But it's not just the fast-food restaurants that are to blame. Macaroni Grill's spaghetti with meatballs and meat sauce serves up 2,430 calories; for that, you could have *nine* hamburgers and a small soda at McDonald's. And not only do these meals give you way too many calories, they're loaded with simple carbohydrates, fat, and salt—a bad combination for anyone, but especially for people who have prediabetes or type 2 diabetes.

Mastering Menus to Manage Diabetes

These alarming calorie and fat counts don't mean you're stuck eating at home and eschewing your favorite splurge meals—you can still enjoy the occasional evening out at a bistro or a weekend diner brunch. If you plan ahead and choose wisely, you won't sacrifice your health by eating out. "You can't live your life to manage a disease, so don't stay away from restaurants completely—you'd be missing out on a huge part of life," says Martha Funnell, RN, CDE, a clinical nurse specialist and codirector of the Behavioral, Clinical, and Health Systems Research Core at the University of Michigan Diabetes Research and Training Center. "You just have to make the right choices, and some of those choices will depend on how often you eat out. If you eat out once every 4 months, you can treat yourself a little more." If you eat out more than once a week, on the other hand, you'll need to find foods that fit well into your diabetes-friendly meal plan.

The key is education. If you know what—and how much—you should eat at restaurants, dining out won't undermine your efforts to control diabetes. And remember, not everyone with pre- or type 2 diabetes shares the same nutrition goals. For some, the focus is on weight loss. "One key to preventing your risk factors is getting down to a healthy weight, and a big part of that is reducing calories," says Dr. Kaufman. Other people need to focus more on boosting fiber, while still others need to cut back on salt and fat. When it's time to place your order, keep your specific goals at the forefront of your mind.

Beyond that, here are some specific actions you can take to have your cake and eat it too, so to speak, when you dine out.

■ **TAKE A COURSE IN FOOD 101.** If you do not know the basics of nutrition, figuring out the most sensible choices on a menu can be as difficult as taking a calculus test without studying. The first thing you should do if you have pre-diabetes or type 2 diabetes is take a crash course in healthy eating. "Go to a diabetes education class or sit down with a nutritionist; once you know about food, you can even eat at McDonald's or Burger King because you will know to order a salad or a BK Broiler," says Donna Rice, RN, CDE, past president of the American Association of Diabetes Educators. "It is all about the decisions you make—you are a product of what you eat."

■ **SAVE RESTAURANTS FOR SPECIAL OCCASIONS.** If you eat out often for business or convenience, the meals are less deserving of a splurge, says Cheryl Marco, RD, CDE, a registered dietitian in the weight management program at Thomas Jefferson University in Philadelphia. If you eat out often and can control yourself in front of a menu, fine. But if you can't shake the "what the heck—I'm out for dinner!" mind-set, then limit yourself to a few outings a month.

■ **CHOOSE ONLY ONE CARBOHYDRATE.** From the moment you sit down at a restaurant, you'll be tempted by simple carbohydrates—a full basket of bread and butter; oversize sides of rice and potatoes; heaping plates of pasta; and so many desserts, they require a separate menu. To avoid sending your blood sugar through the roof, limit yourself to just one carb, Marco says. If you're partial to bread, have it, but skip the rice, potato, and dessert. "If you love sweets, then have a protein [chicken, lean meat, or fish], double up on your vegetables, and save your carbohydrates for dessert—create a balance," she says.

■ **GO FOR BUY ONE, GET ONE FREE.** "Many meals at restaurants are 1,600 calories or more in and of themselves, and that doesn't include a beverage or dessert," says Dr. Marcus. So turn your meal into dinner *and* lunch for the next day. Ask the server to wrap up half of your meal immediately, so you don't even get the chance to polish off your plate.

■ **BEWARE OF BUFFETS.** Buffets are best avoided if you're trying to control diabetes. "Studies have shown that when people go to buffets, they eat more than they would if they were sitting down and being served," says Barry J. Goldstein, MD, PhD, director of the division of endocrinology, diabetes, and metabolic diseases at Jefferson Medical College of Thomas Jefferson University in Philadelphia. If you do find yourself faced with an endless array of options, first pile your plate with salad so there's very little space left for

PLANNING AHEAD IF YOU TAKE MEDS

If you take medication to help control your diabetes, you will need to plan ahead for what and when you will eat. Here are some suggestions from the American Diabetes Association.

- ■ If possible, ask to meet your dinner partners at your normal mealtime.

- ■ Make a reservation (and be on time), and avoid the busiest times for restaurants so you won't have to wait long for your food.

- ■ If you must eat breakfast or lunch later than usual, have a piece of fruit or a starch (such as a slice of whole-grain bread) at your regular mealtime.

- ■ For a late dinner, eat your bedtime snack at your normal mealtime, then eat a full meal at the restaurant. This may require adjusting your insulin.

other foods. Fortunately for you, salads usually come first in line because the ingredients are cheaper. Filling up with low-calorie greens before you get to the other offerings will make you less likely to overeat. A good rule of thumb: Fill half your plate with greens or vegetables, a quarter of it with protein, and a quarter with carbohydrates.

■ **DRESS FOR SUCCESS.** If you top your salad with a vinegar-based dressing, you'll be in even better shape. "Having some kind of acid, such as vinegar, with a meal slows gastric emptying and lowers the glycemic index," says Ralph Felder, MD, PhD, section chief for cardiovascular nutrition, cardiology fellowship program at Banner Good Samaritan Medical Center in Phoenix and author of the *Bonus Years Diet*. Make sure you always order or place dressing on the side so you can control how much goes on your greens.

■ **WHITE OUT YOUR OMELET.** "If you love eggs, egg whites are a great option, and most restaurants will make egg white omelets," says Edwidge Jourdain Thomas, DrNP, assistant professor of clinical nursing at Columbia University. Not only are egg whites low in carbohydrates and cholesterol, they are high in protein and can easily be mixed with broccoli, spinach, and other vegetables, giving you a great start in the morning. "If you can't get past the idea of white eggs, ask the restaurant for a three-egg omelet—one whole egg and the rest whites," she says.

■ **KEEP YOUR WATER GLASS BOTTOM'S UP.** Not only will drinking lots of water at a restaurant keep you hydrated—which is important if you have prediabetes or type 2 diabetes—it will make you full faster. "Sensors in your body let your brain know that you are full and tell you to stop eating," Dr. Thomas says. "Water helps activate those sensors."

■ **KEEP WINE GOBLETS AND BEER STEINS UPRIGHT.** "Drink responsibly" applies to everyone, but even more so if you have prediabetes or type 2 diabetes. "Alcohol is not your friend, caloriewise, when you are watching your weight, and it lowers your inhibitions so you eat more," Dr. Thomas says. "Plus, if you are on medication, alcohol will compete with your liver as far as metabolism is concerned." If you want to have a drink with dinner, keep it to an absolute minimum—one if you're a woman, two if you're a man. And select drinks that are lower in alcohol and sugar. The American Diabetes Association suggests you choose light beer, dry wine, or hard liquor with a sugar-free mixer such as diet soda, diet tonic, club soda, seltzer, or water.

■ **DON'T DRINK ON AN EMPTY STOMACH.** Alcohol slows the release of sugar by the liver, lowering blood sugar. This can be a good thing if you combine a nice glass of red wine with a plate of pasta, but not if you have a few drinks without eating first. In fact, as little as 2 ounces of alcohol on an empty stomach can lead to dangerously low blood sugar levels. "If you are going to drink, combine it with some food," says Rice. "If you order drinks before dinner and the food takes a while to arrive, monitor your blood sugar."

■ **SWEAR OFF FRIED FOODS.** Not only are fried foods loaded with fat and calories, which can pack on extra pounds quickly, they serve up simple carbohydrates in the breading—not a good combination for people concerned about diabetes. "So if you want to have seafood, which is terrific, make sure it is broiled, steamed, or pan-fried—not deep-fried," says Dr. Felder. Also scan the menu for baked, grilled, roasted, or poached items. And keep in mind that menus won't always specify that crab cakes, a Buffalo chicken sandwich, or other dishes will be fried—so ask before you order, or peel off any breading and set it aside.

■ **LET VEGETABLES STEAL THE SHOW.** If your entrée comes with a baked potato or rice pilaf, ask if you can sub a side of steamed vegetables, Dr. Kaufman suggests. Be sure to specify steamed; the usual vegetable sides, such as mixed vegetables or green beans amandine, are often laden with added oils and fats. If side dishes aren't included, order a plate of steamed vegetables anyway and eat them in between bites of your entrée. And box up half of your entrée to take home; otherwise, you may consume too many calories.

■ **DON'T DENY YOURSELF DESSERT.** But share. Just a bite or two might satisfy your sweet tooth, and sharing a piece of cheesecake or a brownie sundae with others at the table will minimize your portion. No one wants to split a decadent dessert with you? Go with a more sensible choice, such as fresh fruit or sorbet. Or order a piece of pie and just eat the fruit—not the crust.

Environmental Exposure

■ **WHAT'S WRONG:** I've been in contact with arsenic, dioxins, or other pesticides and industrial pollutants.

■ **WHY IT MATTERS:** Some studies hint at a possible connection between certain industrial chemicals and diabetes onset. Furthermore, environmental factors may complicate an existing case of diabetes.

■ **THE GOOD NEWS:** The evidence of the connection between these chemicals and diabetes is uncertain and far less of a concern than more preventable factors such as poor diet, a sedentary lifestyle, and obesity. What's more, the environmental factors that can aggravate an existing case are easily controlled through several practical measures.

MAKE NO MISTAKE ABOUT IT—our knowledge of diabetes has grown by leaps and bounds in recent years. Thanks to the hard work of doctors, nutritionists, and other researchers, we have learned much about type 2 diabetes, the type that afflicts 90 to 95 percent of the diabetic population. Meanwhile, type 1 still remains largely mysterious—and some researchers suspect outside influences may affect what's happening within your body.

"Type 1 diabetes occurs because of an autoimmune attack on the body's beta cells, the insulin-producing cells in the pancreas," says Narinder Duggal, MD, an attending physician at Harrison Memorial Hospital in Bremerton, Washington, and medical director of Liberty Bay Internal Medicine in

Poulsbo, Washington. "But we don't know why this attack happens. One theory is that when you have a cold or flu, your body produces antibodies to that virus, as well as antibodies that kill off your body's beta cells."

Meanwhile, another theory holds that environmental factors are partly to blame. "Initial reports suggest that nitrates, nitrites, and related compounds contained in foods and fertilizers might be related to the development of type 1 diabetes," says Beverly Caskey, RPh, a Medco pharmacist who specializes in diabetes care.

Additional evidence indicates that some environmental factors may work with lifestyle factors to hasten the development of type 2 diabetes. "One study found an increase of type 2 diabetes for people living in an area of Italy that had heavy exposure to dioxins due to a 1976 industrial accident," says Caskey. "Arsenic has also been possibly linked with type 2 diabetes."

There's no lack of literature to support these claims. The *Journal of Nutrition,* for example, has published a number of articles suggesting that many of the health concerns in Third World nations, including an increased risk of diabetes, may be associated with high levels of arsenic in drinking water. In 2006, *Environmental Health Perspectives* published a review of numerous studies that looked at the connection between dioxins and diabetes, including studies of factory workers in the states of Missouri and New Jersey and the countries of Germany and Italy, as well as soldiers in the Vietnam War, all whose work exposed them to dioxins. The authors concluded that there may indeed be an association between dioxin exposure and the development of diabetes.

Flaws in the Findings

Many experts remain skeptical about the suggested link between environmental factors and diabetes. The research contains a number of inherent flaws, says David R. Donnersberger, MD, a clinical instructor at Northwestern University Feinberg School of Medicine in Evanston, Illinois. "The studies undoubtedly show that some populations exposed to chemicals have also developed diabetes, but there's no causal relationship between the two," he says. "There's nothing that indicates that high levels of arsenic or other chemicals will do anything to the body's insulin receptors or to insulin resistance."

These chemicals do cause a myriad of problems, but the least of them is a slight, unsubstantiated association with diabetes, says Dr. Donnersberger: "You would have to feed lab mice a large amount of arsenic to see any association with diabetes, and those mice would develop a lot of other problems first." One of the *Journal of Nutrition* studies of arsenic linked the chemical with gastroenteritis, neurological problems, blood vessel changes, and various cancers, as well as diabetes.

Another reason our experts put environmental factors low on the list of risk factors: The known causes of diabetes—poor diet, sedentary lifestyle, and obesity—so greatly outweigh any risks posed by chemicals that they almost render them a nonissue. "People always talk about the link between smoking and lung cancer," says Dr. Duggal. "But if you're obese, you have a greater risk of developing diabetes than a smoker does of developing lung cancer. I'd say that's a pretty significant risk."

Finally, our experts point out that, while still a large concern in the Third World, exposure to these pollutants is becoming increasingly rare in the United States. "A lot of the arsenic exposure is from contaminated drinking water in other parts of the world," says Caskey. "Most water in the United States is routinely monitored for contaminants by state health agencies."

Environmental Aggressors

Though the jury is still out on environmental causes of diabetes, the high risk of complications posed by environmental factors such as extreme cold, high heat, and poor air quality is pretty clear. People with diabetes have a tough time regulating body temperature, which means bitter cold raises their risk of hypothermia and frostbite, while high heat makes them vulnerable to heat exhaustion or heat stroke. "Patients with diabetes have a harder time responding to extra stresses," says Caskey, "and extreme heat places a lot of stress on the body. In addition, sweat caused by this heat may increase the chance for skin infections."

Air irritants pose an additional risk for infection-prone people with diabetes. "Things like smog, smoke, dust, and mold can get into the lungs and cause respiratory infections, as well as other severe problems," says Dr. Donnersberger.

How to Make the Earth Friendly

When you have diabetes, sometimes it can feel like the world has turned against you. Thankfully, that's not the case. By making intelligent choices about how you do—and don't—interact with your surroundings, you can end any environmental issues related to diabetes.

■ **STAMP OUT STRESS.** Amid all the talk of weight loss, exercise, and eating a healthy diet, the role of stress management in diabetes control often takes a backseat. Yet Dr. Duggal says that you can't underestimate its importance.

"Stress is one of the most under-recognized aggravators of diabetes," he says. "When you experience stress, your body releases cortisol, which in turn causes high blood sugar."

In fact, one of the main reasons some people with diabetes struggle with environmental factors is due to the stress they put on the body, adds Dr. Duggal. Read on for ways to control or avoid these environmental stressors.

■ **TEST THE (WELL) WATER.** In the United States, most tap water is frequently monitored and tested for contaminants, so you can be relatively confident that it's safe to drink. "However, untested well water could be a source of arsenic," says Caskey. She recommends having your well water tested regularly by a state or local health official to determine its safety. For a list of state organizations that test water, go to epa.gov/safewater/labs or call 800-426-4791.

■ **AVOID HAZARDOUS ENVIRONMENTS.** The link between diabetes and various pollutants, industrial chemicals, or pesticides may be uncertain, but it's still wise to tread lightly around them. "There may still be other health issues such as cancer, respiratory issues, and reproductive concerns, so make every effort to protect yourself from any unwarranted exposure," such as at the workplace, says Caskey. "Use safety equipment, gloves, masks, and respirators if needed. Encourage your company to continue to find ways to keep everyone safe."

■ **BEAT THE HEAT.** On an extremely hot day, check the news to make sure there's not a heat advisory in your area. If there is, spend the day in an air-conditioned room or building, if possible. A cool shower or bath can also help you regulate your body temperature. If you have to go outside, keep cooler in lightweight, light-colored, and loose-fitting clothing.

■ **STAY IN ON BAD AIR DAYS.** Avoid spending time outdoors if your city's air quality index (AQI) warns that the air is unhealthy that day. Close your windows, and set your air conditioner to recirculate. Try to avoid traffic, where the air quality can be the worst, or outdoor exercise near busy roads—if you're breathing harder during your workout, you'll inhale more irritants.

■ **BE READY TO FACE THE ELEMENTS.** If you do need to go outside on a hot, cold, or bad air day, prime your body to handle the harsh environment. "Diabetics are immuno-compromised, so they need to be aware of the risks and adjust their routines accordingly," says Dr. Donnersberger. "If you're going to be outside on a hot day, drink plenty of water, and take in extra carbohydrates and calories to account for what you'll be losing due to the weather."

■ **STAMP OUT SMOKING.** Of course, being indoors doesn't guarantee safety from air irritants. One of the great risks for anyone—particularly someone with diabetes—is exposure to secondhand tobacco smoke. Caskey recommends instituting a smoking ban inside your home and avoiding other indoor spaces where smoking is allowed, such as bars or restaurants.

■ **SNIFF OUT SAFER PRODUCTS.** Smoking may be the worst violator, but it's not the only indoor air offender. If you have any remodeling or home improvement projects on the horizon, take great care in choosing the paint, glue, and building materials that come into your home. Nearly every product category now has options that are low in volatile organic compounds (VOCs), which make them better for the Earth and better for your body. And decorate with live plants: "They are nature's air purifiers," says Caskey.

■ **PRACTICE DIABETES BASICS.** Controlling your environment may help keep diabetes symptoms in check, but it still plays second fiddle to other concerns for diabetes management. "Whereas many environmental factors are a matter of circumstance, lifestyle choices have been shown to prevent or improve diabetes outcomes," says Caskey. "Concentrate on the areas that truly make a difference: Eat healthy foods; exercise; maintain a healthy weight; and keep blood sugar, blood pressure, and cholesterol under control."

Lack of Exercise

■ **WHAT'S WRONG:** I spend most of the time sitting, whether it's on the sofa, behind my desk, or in a car.

■ **WHY IT MATTERS:** Regular exercise can prevent prediabetes from turning into diabetes. It may also help you lower your blood sugar with less medication, and it can help prevent the serious complications of diabetes. In fact, some experts call it a magic pill.

■ **THE GOOD NEWS:** One study found that people with diabetes who walked regularly had a 39 percent lower risk of dying from their disease. Another estimated that for each 61 people who walked at least 2 hours a week, one death a year would be prevented!

WHEN PEOPLE WHO ARE NEWLY DIAGNOSED with diabetes walk into Gary Scheiner's office, he tries to give them a message they can't ignore. "I say, 'I'm not a religious person, but if there's such a thing as God's wake-up call, this is it. This is your chance to take better care of your body. If you don't do it, God's taking it back,'" says Scheiner, an exercise physiologist, certified diabetes educator, and owner of Integrated Diabetes Services in Wynnewood, Pennsylvania. He's also had diabetes for 24 years and relies on physical activity as a cornerstone for managing his blood sugar.

If clients don't find that message motivating enough, he may toss another their way: "This is your opportunity to get yourself into good shape. Or keep doing what you're doing and go downhill. The type 2 diabetic who doesn't exercise is just asking to die of a premature—and grisly—death."

Although people with diabetes may generally know that exercise—and just being generally active—is good for them, many simply don't do it enough, exercise experts say. "Sometimes when we're presenting information to a class of new patients who have just been diagnosed, they get this glazed look on their faces. A lot of them are getting their diets and medications regulated, then somebody says, 'Guess what's really going to help you . . . moving!' They're not real receptive at first," says Jennifer Hopper, manager of the Piedmont Hospital Health and Fitness Club in Atlanta.

One reason people may not be excited about jumping into an exercise program is because they've heard that they need at least 30 minutes of exercise most days to stay healthy. Before they can even fathom doing that much, they may learn that some experts now advise *60* minutes of exercise daily, and that sounds even more impossible, says Sheri Colberg, PhD, a diabetes author and associate professor of exercise science at Old Dominion University in Norfolk, Virginia. The groups making the stepped-up recommendations "forget that the people weren't even doing the 30 minutes, and they make people say, 'Heck, I'm not going to do that, so why bother?'" she says.

Other people with diabetes may take the opposite approach by trying to become too active too quickly. They might be able to keep up their new habits for a while, but their resolve dwindles, and they feel like failures because they can't keep up their new routines. Or they get injured and never get back into the groove. Whatever the reason, they stop exercising . . . which isn't good because their diabetes is going to remain a problem for the rest of their lives, and exercise needs to be a lifelong treatment.

Can't seem to find inspiration to get your muscles pumping? Look to Bob Cleveland for motivation. In her book, *50 Secrets of the Longest Living People with Diabetes*, Dr. Colberg interviewed a variety of people who'd been controlling their diabetes for decades to glean what worked best for them. Cleveland, who'd had diabetes for more than 80 years when he talked to Dr. Colberg, said, "Probably my number one secret is to be physically active. I can't walk very well anymore, but I'll go out and ride my bike 20 miles at a time."

Dr. Colberg says, "If I could have, I would have jumped over the phone and given that guy a kiss and said, 'That's the right answer!'"

The message Scheiner, Hopper, Dr. Colberg, and other exercise professionals with an interest in diabetes want to offer is this: Becoming more physically active protects your body and mind in many, many ways when you have diabetes. Not only is it crucial for keeping your blood sugar in control now, it can help prevent a host of serious problems later. It can improve not only the quantity but the quality of your life. And gently and gradually easing your way into more physical activity is the best way to make it a long-term habit.

"If there were a magic pill that could make you happy, provide you with an opportunity to lose weight—that could lower your blood pressure, reduce cholesterol, and improve your sleep—that's exercise," Hopper says. "It's that magic pill."

Let's take a look at how exercise can make controlling your blood sugar easier now and prevent bad things from happening to you for decades to come. Lacing up your exercise shoes may seem far easier when you know the benefits it brings. (See Make Exercise an Everyday Event on page 314 to learn just how to make exercise part of your daily routine.)

Exercise: The Right Move for Preventing and Controlling Diabetes

Exercise can play a key role in limiting the effect that diabetes will have on your life even before you develop the disease. A landmark 2002 study called the Diabetes Prevention Program highlighted the effects of physical activity in people who were overweight and had a type of prediabetes. The researchers found that people who lost 7 percent of their body weight by improving their diets and exercising 150 minutes a week (that's just 2½ hours) lowered their risk of developing diabetes by 58 percent. Others in the study took the blood-sugar-lowering drug metformin twice a day and lowered their risk by a lesser amount—31 percent.

Most people with prediabetes go on to develop diabetes within 10 years if they don't lose weight with lifestyle changes, according to the National Institutes of Health. They also face a higher risk of heart disease. So if you know that you have prediabetes or other risk factors for developing diabetes, don't wait until you have the disease to start becoming more active. The health benefits start now!

If you already have diabetes, being more physically active will provide major health benefits, both immediately and over the long term.

■ **YOU'LL GAIN BETTER BLOOD SUGAR CONTROL.** An essential problem of diabetes is that your blood glucose is too high. For people with type 1 diabetes, that's because the pancreas stops making insulin, which must be present in your blood to allow cells in your muscles and other tissues to let in blood glucose for fuel. In type 2 diabetes, your cells become resistant to insulin—they essentially ignore it—and your pancreas pumps out more of the hormone. Eventually, though, it starts producing less and less of it. People with early type 2 diabetes may have 40 percent less glucose uptake into their cells, compared with people without diabetes.

A single session of aerobic exercise—whole-body, heart-pumping activities like biking and walking—can make your body more sensitive to insulin for 24 to 72 hours, depending on the length and intensity of your workout. That's at least a day for your cells to gobble up more glucose and get it out of your bloodstream, where it may be causing damage to tissues all over your body.

As a result, for type 2 diabetes in particular, exercise is "an absolute necessity" for blood sugar control, Scheiner says. The research backs it up. In one meta-analysis—in which a researcher compiles previous studies to produce a big-picture measurement—people who took part in structured exercise for at least 8 weeks had more than half a percentage point lower A1C, a common test that measures overall blood sugar control over the past few months.

Half a percentage point might not sound like much . . . until you consider that research has found that each percentage-point reduction in A1C is associated with a 21 percent lower risk of dying from diabetes, 14 percent lower risk of heart attack, and 37 percent lower risk of complications in small blood vessels (the underlying cause of complications such as retina damage in the eyes).

Strength-training exercise—such as lifting weights—has also been found to aid blood sugar control. Two studies involving people with type 2 diabetes who were mostly in their 60s found that those who did high-intensity strength training three times a week saw their A1C drop by more than 1 percentage point, compared with people who didn't do the exercise program. Other research on strength training that involved less-intense workouts also found helpful effects.

Keeping your blood sugar controlled is the name of the game in diabetes, and exercise will help you do it. But it may also help you avoid needing meds for management, Scheiner says. "I've had a lot of patients who have been able to get off insulin and other medications because they embraced exercise and lost weight and made some changes in their lifestyles," he says. "No one likes medications, and they certainly don't like taking insulin if they can help it. The opportunity to eliminate or cut down on those is motivating." You shouldn't change your medication regimen without your doctor's okay, but as you shed pounds and get your blood sugar lower, your doctor eventually may agree that you can cut out some pills or injections.

■ **YOU'LL WHITTLE YOUR MIDDLE.** Losing weight also helps decrease insulin resistance—that problem when your cells "ignore" the hormone, stranding blood sugar out in your bloodstream. You don't even have to lose much to see these improvements—dropping just 10 percent of your body weight can do it. According to the American College of Sports Medicine (ACSM), losing weight might be most helpful to diabetes control earlier in the process, when your pancreas is still pumping out enough insulin.

Research has found that exercise is especially good for trimming fat around your midsection. The fat inside your abdomen—called visceral fat—is particularly bad for your blood sugar. As it increases, your insulin sensitivity goes down. "What's really interesting is that the best way to lose that really bad fat inside your abdomen is through physical activity—it's not through dieting," Dr. Colberg says. "Dieting plus exercise works, but what works best is just the exercise."

A 2007 study in the journal *Diabetes Care* reported the results of a major study involving more than 5,000 middle-aged and older overweight people with type 2 diabetes. People assigned to an intensive lifestyle-changing program—which involved losing just 7 percent of their weight, a restricted-calorie diet, and working toward 175 minutes of exercise weekly—saw many big benefits.

Compared with people who merely received a few diabetes-education sessions, the first group lost more weight (8.6 percent versus 0.7 percent), had a bigger A1C drop (7.3 to 6.6 percent versus 7.3 to 7.2 percent), and saw significantly bigger improvements in their blood pressure, triglycerides, and HDL cholesterol.

According to the ACSM's position statement on exercise and type 2 diabetes, one of the factors that's most strongly associated with long-term weight control is how much exercise you do. You're going to have diabetes for the rest of your life (or be at higher risk of it if you have prediabetes), so you should strive to maintain your weight loss for the long haul.

Experts say that you probably need at least five 1-hour sessions of exercise each week to keep the weight off long-term—but don't let that scare you. As you'll see in Part IV, all you have to do right now is get started. Once you dip your toe in the water and make exercise a little part of your life, you may gradually find that you don't even mind doing it more often.

■ **YOU'LL PRESERVE FAT-BURNING MUSCLE.** Although you want to lose excess fat, you definitely don't want to lose valuable muscle, but that's exactly what happens to many people as they get older. After you turn 30, you lose about 3 to 8 percent of your muscle mass each decade, and the loss speeds up after age 60. That's bad news for blood sugar control on two fronts. Your muscles are like your body's calorie-burning furnaces: As they dwindle, your body burns fewer calories each day. If you keep eating the same amount of calories, you'll start to put on more fat—mostly the superbad kind deep in your abdomen, Dr. Colberg warns. In addition, with less muscle mass, your body responds less well to its insulin supply.

Although strength training is the type of exercise that most people probably associate with preserving their muscles, aerobic exercise is helpful, too.

■ **YOU'LL KEEP BLOOD PRESSURE STEADY.** Roughly two-thirds of adults with diabetes also have high blood pressure, presenting a double whammy to their health. If you have both problems, you're at even higher risk of diabetes complications such as heart disease, stroke, eye problems, and kidney damage.

A 2005 study from the *Archives of Internal Medicine* that looked at 2,316 men with diabetes (average age: 50) found that normal-weight, overweight, and obese guys who were unfit were all roughly 2.7 times more likely to die of a cardiovascular cause than fit guys of normal weight. Losing weight is a good idea, but don't hold off on exercise until you can get down to a certain weight—and don't give up on it just because you aren't dropping down to your dream weight fast enough. The practice is still doing you good. "The importance of avoiding a sedentary lifestyle and a low fitness level by individuals with diabetes cannot be overstated," the authors write—and there's no reason these benefits of staying fit wouldn't apply to women, too.

Even if you don't have diabetes yet, high blood pressure may be a special concern for you. Roughly 50 million Americans have a condition called metabolic syndrome, according to the American Heart Association. This is marked by a variety of issues including obesity carried around the abdomen, high blood pressure, and insulin resistance or glucose intolerance. It puts you at higher risk of heart disease, stroke, and type 2 diabetes. The AHA recommends that the first steps toward reducing those health-threatening factors are to lose weight if you're overweight and get physical activity on most days of the week.

If you have diabetes, you should aim to keep your blood pressure below 130/80 mm Hg (millimeters of mercury), according to the AHA. Thirty minutes of exercise on most days of the week—even broken into 10-minute chunks—is important for controlling or preventing high blood pressure, according to the National Institutes of Health.

■ **YOU'LL TAKE CONTROL OF YOUR CHOLESTEROL.** Some research has found that people with type 2 diabetes who participate in physical activity can see improvements in their triglycerides, total cholesterol, and ratio of "good"

HDL to "bad" LDL cholesterol. This may help reduce your risk of atherosclerosis, the process through which plaque accumulates in your arteries, setting the stage for heart disease or stroke.

■ **YOU'LL BOOST YOUR MOOD AND MIND.** Depression is a major problem for people with diabetes, Dr. Colberg points out, and along with day-to-day stress can keep you from maintaining good diabetes control. Exercise addresses both of these issues.

"I think for that reason alone—the mental-health benefits—I've kept with my exercise all these years," says Dr. Colberg, who's had type 1 diabetes since she was 4 years old. "Physical or emotional stress wreaks havoc on your diabetes control, and one of the best ways to help control your emotional stress is through physical activity. Exercise is also one of the most natural treatments for mild to moderate depression."

In addition, exercise may help keep your mind sharp. People with diabetes face a higher risk of Alzheimer's disease and vascular dementia (mental difficulties caused by lack of blood flow to the brain), Dr. Colberg says. A 2007 study from Sweden found that even "borderline" diabetes was associated with a 67 and 77 percent greater chance of developing dementia and Alzheimer's, respectively. The higher levels of insulin in your body that accompany insulin resistance may promote inflammation and other problems in your brain that set the stage for Alzheimer's, other research has found.

The people in their 80s and 90s whom Dr. Colberg spoke to for her book had "no sign" of Alzheimer's, she said. Exercise can help keep the blood-carrying arteries to your brain clear of plaques, and the better-controlled insulin and blood sugar may make you less likely to develop Alzheimer's.

Lack of Sleep

■ **WHAT'S WRONG:** I get less than 7 hours of sleep a night.

■ **WHY IT MATTERS:** Sleeping too little (or too much) can elevate insulin levels.

■ **THE GOOD NEWS:** Because sleep plays such an important role in metabolic control, getting just the right amount of rest each night could support weight management and blood sugar balance.

MORE PEOPLE THAN EVER are getting by on just a few hours of shut-eye. Whether the reason is insomnia or lifestyle trends, up to 20 percent of women regularly clock in fewer than 5 hours of rest a night. And in a survey by the Better Sleep Council, a nonprofit organization in Alexandria, Virginia, nearly 70 percent of women between ages 40 and 60 reported getting fewer than 8 hours a night. You may have heard that it's normal to sleep less when you get older. But just because we get less sleep doesn't mean we need less as we age.

"Our bodies want rest," says Michael V. Vitiello, PhD, professor of psychiatry and behavioral sciences at the University of Washington in Seattle. "We just can't generate it like we once did." Natural changes in aging neurons alter the quantity and quality of our sleep, and sleep problems such as insomnia, restless legs syndrome (aching, tingling, or discomfort in the calves), and sleep apnea (heavy snoring and interrupted breathing) are more common when we're over 40.

These conditions can keep you from getting your optimum 7 to 8 hours of sleep. But even if you're sleeping less by choice, you might want to reconsider, especially if you have type 2 diabetes or are at risk for it.

It's no surprise that the trend toward sleeping less coincides with the dramatic increases in obesity and diabetes, say researchers at the University of Chicago. They recently reported that people who slept fewer than 5 hours a night were $2\frac{1}{2}$ times more likely to develop diabetes than those who got 7 to 8 hours of rest.

If that isn't enough to stress you out, the Chicago researchers also found that inadequate shut-eye may cause levels of the stress hormone cortisol to spike in the afternoon and evening—increasing heart rate, blood pressure, and blood glucose. Aside from posing future health problems, the cortisol-induced alertness comes at an inopportune time—when you should be winding down your day or sleeping.

Skimping on sleep can also increase hunger and impair glucose tolerance, even in healthy people. That's because lack of sleep triggers the hunger-inducing hormone ghrelin and lowers the appetite-suppressing hormone leptin. So you

NAVIGATING THE NIGHT SHIFT

Are you working into the wee hours when you'd rather be sleeping? Your body wasn't designed to work the night shift or rotating shifts. But if you have no choice, follow these strategies to steer clear of sleeplessness.

- Use bright lights to mimic daylight to keep you awake.

- Try to stay on the same shift, but if you must rotate, do it by the clock: from days to afternoons to nights.

- If you can't sleep when you get home in the morning, don't force it. Wait till early afternoon when you have an energy dip.

crave more calories than your body needs, especially in the form of sugary snacks and starches. Sleeping less than 6 hours a night also raises your insulin levels, which can make you crave fatty foods. "This may explain why sleep-deprived people often have trouble losing weight," says Sara C. Mednick, PhD, a research scientist at the Salk Institute for Biological Studies in La Jolla, California, and author of *Take a Nap! Change Your Life.*

On the flip side, sleeping too much—9 hours or more a night—may triple your odds of getting diabetes, even in the absence of other risk factors, according to a Yale University study of 1,709 men. Previous studies have turned up similar findings in women. When you sleep either too little or too long, your nervous system stays on alert and interferes with hormones that regulate blood sugar, says lead researcher Klar Yaggi, MD, assistant professor of pulmonary medicine at the Yale School of Medicine.

Understanding all the ways sleep affects diabetes can be confusing because the data are so intertwined, says Helene A. Emsellem, MD, director of the Center for Sleep and Wake Disorders in Chevy Chase, Maryland, and author of *Snooze . . . or Lose!: 10 "No-War" Ways to Improve Your Teen's Sleep Habits.* If you're having trouble sleeping, you're more likely to have trouble controlling your blood sugar; but if your blood sugar is out of control, you're more likely to have trouble falling asleep and you'll be sleepier during the day. Which comes first? There's data in both directions, Dr. Emsellem says.

While your odds of suffering from sleep apnea and restless legs syndrome increase with age, having diabetes also increases your risk. "At least 25 percent of people with diabetes also have RLS, which may be caused in part by peripheral neuropathy as a complication of diabetes," Dr. Emsellem says. Both sleep apnea and RLS disturb the quality of your sleep, so you may end up oversleeping or getting sleepy during the day.

Being overweight also increases your risk for sleep apnea—and for diabetes. But even if you're not overweight, diabetes increases your risk of having sleep apnea. If you're not sleeping enough, or you sleep too long because of RLS or apnea, you're more likely to gain weight, which increases your risk of developing diabetes. See the problem? It's a crazy catch-22.

The best strategy is to keep a tight rein on your blood sugar in general, which should help you sleep. At the same time, treat any sleep disorders. That way you can make the most of your 8 hours in the land of nod, which in turn should help you control your diabetes. "Everything falls back to tighter diabetes control," explains Dr. Emsellem. "Sleep is a factor in controlling your blood sugar, weight is clearly a factor in controlling your blood sugar, and sleep is a factor in controlling your weight."

Are You a Healthy Sleeper?

To find out, check off any of the statements that apply to you.

- I regularly take at least 30 minutes to fall asleep.

- I snore, gasp, or snort loudly and regularly during the night.

- Most nights, I wake up and can't fall back asleep.

- I generally do not wake up feeling refreshed.

- My legs regularly twitch during the night.

- I tend to nod off at inappropriate times, such as during business meetings.

- I get less than 6 hours of actual sleep.

- I stay in bed for 9 hours or more.

If you checked just one of the above statements, talk to your doctor about screening for sleep apnea, RLS, or another medical condition, such as depression, that might be cutting into your sleep schedule.

If you have RLS, your doctor will most likely prescribe a specific medication to control the condition. If you have mild sleep apnea, a dental jaw advancement appliance may help you breathe easier. Losing weight can also help reduce symptoms. For more severe sleep apnea, your doctor may recommend that you wear a device called CPAP (continuous positive airway pressure) when you sleep.

In addition, ask your doctor if any medications you're taking might be causing insomnia as a side effect. If so, you might need a medicine cabinet makeover. "Medications that treat cardiovascular and respiratory conditions can affect the neurotransmitters involved in sleep," explains Amy Wolfson, PhD, author of *The Woman's Book of Sleep*. And antihistamines and antidepressants can suppress REM sleep—the deep, recuperative stage tied to memory. If your meds are hampering your Zzzs, you may be able to switch drugs or change when you take them.

Here are a few more tips to help you doze away diabetes.

▓ **STICK TO A SCHEDULE.** A regular sleep schedule takes advantage of your circadian rhythm (your internal body clock). "If you have diabetes and you have a job and a family with lots of things going on, you really need to preserve your block of time for sleep," says Dr. Emsellem. Sleeping in on Saturday morning may sound like a good idea, but you're actually setting yourself up for more sleep problems come Monday. With each schedule change, your body has to reset its circadian rhythm, and this fluctuation may hinder restorative rest.

▓ **CUT BACK ON CAFFEINE AFTER 2 P.M.** Coffee isn't the only culprit; colas, chocolate, tea, and some medications also contain caffeine. And skip the nightcap if you're within 3 hours of bedtime. "Drinking alcohol can make you drowsy, but it tends to disrupt sleep in the middle of the night," says Dr. Emsellem.

▓ **STAY HYDRATED.** Even mild dehydration—losing as little as half a cup of body water—could turn into low-grade chronic fatigue. Drink eight to ten 8-ounce glasses of water a day, and add four to six more glasses when you exercise. To prevent unnecessary trips to the bathroom at night, be sure to empty your bladder before going to sleep.

▓ **EAT EARLIER.** Overeating after 8 p.m. not only will keep you awake, it also will channel energy to the digestive process and away from restorative tasks that occur when you're sleeping, says Dr. Emsellem. Instead, eat your largest meals earlier in the day so you can linger over lighter suppers. Avoid feasting on spicy or gassy fare, but have a small bite about an hour before bed to help you fall asleep and keep your stomach from growling.

The Diabetes Lowdown

For years doctors warned people with sleep disorders that taking naps would interfere with nighttime sleep. But the evidence now shows you *can* get to sleep at night, even when you take a nap. Turns out the period in the middle of the day, when we usually feel out of it, is our natural naptime.

"There's a little dip in our circadian rhythm between about 1 and 3 p.m., and we get this little dip in energy in all our processes, including our glucose metabolism and our cortisol," says Sara C. Mednick, PhD, a research scientist at the Salk Institute for Biological Studies in La Jolla, California, and author of *Take a Nap! Change Your Life.* A daytime nap may actually help you sleep better at night because you'll be less likely to reach for caffeine in the afternoon, "which is the real vicious cycle that depletes your sleep," she says.

Taking regular naps may also lower your risk of a serious diabetes complication: heart disease. A recent Harvard University study of more than 23,000 people found that regular nappers lowered their risk of dying from a heart attack by 37 percent. People who took only occasional naps still lowered their risk by 12 percent.

To get the most benefit out of a daytime doze, Dr. Mednick suggests limiting naps to no longer than $1\frac{1}{2}$ hours, ending at least 2 hours before bedtime. "You don't need that long of a nap every day, but a great weekend nap would be perfect, with small 15-minute naps during the week," she says.

■ **WORK OUT TO WIND DOWN.** Regular exercise first energizes, then relaxes you. A vigorous workout right before bed releases nerve-stimulating hormones that will raise your body's core temperature, preventing you from falling asleep. Instead, exercise at least 3 hours before bedtime to put you in cooldown mode just as you hit the sack. This helps induce deep sleep, according to the National Sleep Foundation.

■ **TRY TAI CHI OR YOGA.** You don't have to work up an intense sweat to reap the benefits of exercise. Practicing tai chi three times a week for 6 months can result in longer, more restful sleep, according to a study of 118 people from the Oregon Research Institute in Eugene. Doing Kundalini yoga (a technique that combines meditation, breathing, and postures) for at least half an hour a day for 8 weeks has also been shown to increase sleep by about 36 minutes, say Harvard University researchers.

■ **WALK INTO SLEEP.** Taking a walk may provide the same benefits as taking sleep medication—without the side effects, such as grogginess, increased snoring, risk of sleep apnea, and possible addiction. You don't have to walk far to get sleep-enhancing benefits. People who walked at least six blocks a day at a normal pace were a third less likely to have trouble sleeping, according to one study of more than 700 men and women. Those who picked up the pace had even better sleeping habits.

■ **IF YOU'RE STILL SMOKING, QUIT.** Smoking interferes with different stages of sleep, including REM (rapid eye movement) sleep. A study of 484 people ages 14 to 84 found that smokers were more likely to have daytime sleepiness and consume caffeine than nonsmokers were. Smoking also increases your risk of snoring and sleep apnea, which can disturb your sleep and increase your risk of developing diabetes. While you're trying to quit, you may suffer a few more restless nights, but your sleep quality should soon improve.

■ **LISTEN TO LUDWIG.** A Taiwanese and American study of 60 troubled sleepers found that listening to soft music 45 minutes before bed for 3 weeks improved sleep quality and quantity by 35 percent. The most relaxing music has 60 to 80 beats per minute, such as Beethoven symphonies, Bach preludes, or Bob Dylan folk tunes.

■ **SALUTE THE MORNING SUN.** Taking a 10-minute stroll before your morning cup of decaf may help reset your wake-sleep cycle. Studies suggest getting a little sunshine early in the day can help your body produce nighttime melatonin, the hormone that regulates sleep.

■ **NIX THE NIGHT-LIGHTS.** Exposure to the bright, concentrated glow of a television or computer screen less than 1 hour before bedtime is enough light to upset your circadian rhythm and delay sleep. Any light signals the brain to wake up, but "blue light" from your cell phone and your clock's digital display are the worst offenders. For a sound sleep, turn off the TV, turn your clock around, and banish blinking Blackberrys, computers, and other lighted devices from the bedroom.

■ **TALK YOURSELF TO SLEEP.** Instead of taking sleeping pills, consider counseling. In one 8-week-long study, cognitive-behavioral therapy helped 33 insomniacs alter negative thinking ("I'm never going to fall asleep") and develop better sleep habits, such as limiting their time spent in bed to sleep and sex only. It may not sound like much, but researchers at Harvard Medical School and Beth Israel Deaconess Medical Center found the therapy to be 30 percent more effective than drugs in treating insomnia.

■ **SLIP ON SOME SOCKS.** The instant warm-up widens blood vessels in your feet, allowing your body to transfer heat from its core to the extremities, cooling you slightly, which induces sleep, says Phyllis Zee, PhD, director of sleep disorders at Northwestern University's Feinberg School of Medicine.

■ **PERFECT YOUR NIGHTTIME POSTURE.** Try these sleep positions for a more restful night.

- To relieve lower-back pressure, try putting a pillow under your knees. The pillow comfortably flexes your lower spine.

- To avoid neck and shoulder aches, rest your head on a pillow made with down instead of foam. Choose a pillow low enough to support your head without flexing your neck. If you have chronic neck problems, try an orthopedic pillow with the middle scooped out.

- To keep warm, pull on a warmer blanket rather than curling up, which can leave you with a sore back.

- To prevent stiff joints, allow yourself enough room to move your arms and legs and roll over during the night.

Overweight

■ **WHAT'S WRONG:** I weigh more than I should.

■ **WHY IT MATTERS:** Overweight contributes to insulin resistance and is a major risk factor for diabetes and its complications.

■ **THE GOOD NEWS:** The Diabetes Prevention Program study showed that losing as little as 5 to 7 percent of your body weight (for most people, about 10 to 15 pounds) and exercising for 150 minutes per week (an average of 30 minutes per day, 5 days a week) can help reduce your risk of diabetes by 58 percent.

A FEW HUNDRED YEARS AGO, being overweight was considered beautiful; after all, if you were carrying some extra pounds, it meant you were wealthy enough to lounge around eating grapes while someone else chased down dinner. And with the average life expectancy being only about 35, people didn't notice the heavy toll that obesity took on blood sugar and overall health.

Today, being overweight is not so fashionable, but it certainly appears popular. The World Health Organization reports that there are more than one billion overweight adults, and at least 300 million of them are classified as obese. The obesity epidemic has even spread to genetically thin countries, such as China and Japan. In this country, 65 percent—more than half!—of Americans are overweight, 30 percent are obese, and the problem is putting on more weight every day.

Despite the current media's portrayal of thin as in, why are so many people overweight? The simple answer: because of diets high in fat and sugar combined with sedentary lifestyles. If you look more deeply, it is because of the evolution from a hunter-and-gatherer culture to our current lifestyles full of modern conveniences. Our ancestors couldn't drive to the nearest grocery store to buy food, so their bodies adapted to be able to live for extended periods without nourishment; in short, they easily put on weight to "store up" for the times when food was scarce. As a result, we have bodies designed to store calories combined with modern conveniences designed to help us avoid activity—a recipe for a society that is overweight.

A Portly Problem for Blood Sugar

This overweight epidemic is a heavy contributor to the increasing rates of prediabetes and type 2 diabetes. More than 20 million adults and children in this country have diabetes (90 to 95 percent of whom have type 2), and another 54 million have prediabetes. Weight loss is so critical for all of these people because there is a direct link between overweight and risk of the disease. "About 85 percent of people with type 2 diabetes or prediabetes are overweight," says Ralph Felder, MD, PhD, section chief for cardiovascular nutrition, cardiology fellowship program at Banner Good Samaritan Medical Center in Phoenix and author of the *Bonus Years Diet*.

The problem is that fat doesn't just sit there making your jeans hard to button. "Fat is actually very metabolically active," says Alan Marcus, MD, a physician in private practice in Laguna Hills, California, who specializes in diabetes management and endocrinology. "Fat produces hormones that interfere with insulin and send out messages to your body to either not respond to insulin or to make more insulin."

Plus, excess weight contributes to even further weight gain because it makes exercise uncomfortable, so you're less likely to move and more likely to put on more pounds. "Weight stops the body from performing what it needs to do to stay healthy—it puts a tremendous strain on the muscles and joints, and it is very important for these muscles and joints to be exercised," Dr. Marcus says. When the body fails to get exercise, it doesn't metabolize glucose as efficiently. "Once glucose occurs in excess in the body, it becomes a poison," he says.

In addition to raising blood sugar, the vicious cycle that goes along with being overweight has many other detrimental effects on the body. "If you are overweight, you become insulin resistant, your cholesterol goes up, high cholesterol propagates insulin resistance, and you may eventually develop diabetes," says Eric Yan, MD, physician nutrition specialist at Valens Medical in Irvine, California.

When they occur together, all the above risk factors are lumped under one label—"metabolic syndrome." Metabolic syndrome—also called syndrome X and the deadly quartet—consists of a combination of abdominal fat, blood pressure higher than 135/85 mm Hg (millimeters of mercury), high cholesterol and triglycerides, and an elevated glucose level. At least one out of every five overweight people has several of these factors at once.

A Little Fat Loss Equals Big Health Benefits

Luckily, no matter if you have 20 pounds to lose or 200, dropping even a small amount of weight will make a major difference in terms of your diabetes risk. "You only have to lose 2.5 percent of your body mass to reverse glucose elevations," Dr. Marcus says. Not only will this minimal weight loss reduce your risk of diabetes, it will improve your blood pressure, cholesterol, and triglyceride levels and decrease inflammation, all of which will lower your risk for heart attack and stroke.

To lose the weight, it seems the old reliable—a combination of diet and exercise—is your best bet. A groundbreaking study called the Diabetes Prevention Program followed 3,234 people with prediabetes. "One-third of the participants received simple instructions about lifestyle, one-third received intensive lifestyle intervention, and the remaining third got treatment with the drug metformin," says Barry J. Goldstein, MD, PhD, director of the division of endocrinology, diabetes, and metabolic diseases at Jefferson Medical College of Thomas Jefferson University in Philadelphia, who worked on the study. "Initial results show that the intensive lifestyle intervention, which included both diet and exercise, was most effective—even more effective than the drug—and delayed the onset of diabetes by 58 percent," he says.

The first step in weight loss—and therefore improved blood sugar levels and overall health—is assessing where you are, where you want to be, and how you plan to get there. Here's how.

■ **CHECK FOR A SPARE TIRE.** It seems that where fat parks itself on your body is at least as important as the number of extra pounds you carry. "Even though you may not like the fact that you have a larger butt and thighs, that fat tends to be less of a determinant of pre- and type 2 diabetes than abdominal fat," says Dr. Goldstein. "Abdominal fat is associated more with an insulin resistance effect on the body."

To find out if you are carrying too much fat around your middle, measure it at its widest point. If your waist is over 35 inches if you are a woman and over 40 inches if you are a man, chances are you are already in the prediabetes category. Another way to determine whether or not you are overweight is by determining your body mass index (BMI). Use the calculator on the Centers for Disease Control and Prevention's Web site: http://www.cdc.gov/nccdphp/dnpa/bmi/index.htm. A BMI of 25 or higher is considered overweight; if it's 30 or over, you are classified as obese.

■ **COMPUTE YOUR CALORIE NEEDS.** Before you begin a weight loss plan, figure out how many pounds you need to lose and how many calories you need to cut to get there. Start by calculating the number of calories you need to take in each day to maintain your weight. Let's suppose you weight 150 pounds. If you are inactive, you require 10 to 11 calories per pound. So you'll maintain your weight if you eat 1,500 calories a day. If you're mildly active, you burn 13 calories per pound, or about 1,950 calories a day. If you are active—you work out for at least 30 to 60 minutes three times a week—you burn 15 calories per pound, or 2,250 calories.

If you're overweight, you probably weigh more than 150. As a rule of thumb, you need a deficit of 3,500 calories to lose 1 pound of body fat. If you cut 250 calories per day—the amount in a chocolate bar or a large soda at a fast-food restaurant—you can lose a half a pound a week. If you cut 500 calories per day, you can lose 1 pound per week.

■ **FIND A MOTIVATOR.** "I tell people to find a daughter they have to marry off; basically, this means that if you have something to commit to, you will lose the weight. Most women who have a daughter who is getting married will try to lose some weight before the wedding," says Fred Vagnini, MD, medical director of the Cardiovascular Wellness Centers of New York in New York City. "Personally, I was obese and I had little kids, so I knew I had to turn myself around." If nothing in your personal life is motivating you, think about the health problems related to being overweight—if you lose just a few pounds, you'll reduce your risk not only for diabetes but for heart attack and stroke. Plus, losing weight will help you look and feel better and give you more energy to do the things you enjoy.

■ **PLAN TO PACE YOURSELF.** When you start to lose weight, it can be tempting to crash diet in order to see results fast. But this strategy will backfire. "If you lose 5 pounds in a week, you will gain another 7 the next week," says Edwidge Jourdain Thomas, DrNP, assistant professor of clinical nursing at Columbia University. "So aim for a weight loss of 1 pound per week. If you combine diet and exercise, you can lose almost 2 pounds per week, but overall, your goal should be 1 pound."

■ **WATCH YOUR WEIGHT.** Literally. "Some overweight people have not gone near a scale in years," says Neal D. Barnard, MD, adjunct associate professor of medicine at George Washington University School of Medicine and Health Services and author of *Dr. Neal Barnard's Program for Reversing Diabetes*. If you fall into this category, invest in a scale so you can track your progress. "And use the same scale each time you weigh yourself—different scales can give you dramatically different readings," Dr. Barnard says.

Once you are ready to begin, follow these tips to lose weight—and as a result, lower your risk for prediabetes or type 2 diabetes and complications of the disease.

Diabetes-Proof Your Diet

"At the end of the day, it is really reducing your total calorie intake in a way that doesn't make you hungry—and still gives you balanced nutrient composition and the necessary vitamins and minerals—that leads to weight loss success," Dr. Goldstein says. "The important advice is to increase intake of fiber, fruits, and vegetables; reduce saturated fat [animal fat found in red meat and full-fat dairy products]; and eat healthier fat calories, like healthy oils [oils found in fish and nuts]." Beyond that:

■ **FORGO FAD DIETS.** If you want to lose weight, forget about losing 20 pounds in 20 days with the latest trendy diet, Dr. Felder says. "And low-carb diets are dangerous because they put you in ketoacidosis [a serious condition that can lead to diabetic coma or even death]. You may lose weight with these diets, but a lot of it is water weight," he says. "Instead, you need to have a balanced diet." To achieve balance, Dr. Felder recommends 4 cups of fruits and vegetables, 2 ounces of nuts, 5 ounces of wine, and a clove of garlic a day, plus fish three times a week.

■ **FILL UP ON FIBER.** In addition to making us more sedentary, modern technology has stripped some of the valuable fiber from our foods. For example, to produce white rice, manufacturers remove its fiber-rich brown coating. "But you are better off if it is left intact," Dr. Barnard says. "Each 14 grams of fiber added to your daily menu cuts calorie intake by about 10 percent, on average. High-fiber foods will fill you up faster, so you stop eating sooner." Healthful high-fiber foods include beans, vegetables, fruits, and whole grains. Veggies are a particularly good way to get fiber because they'll fill you up with few calories. Aim for a total of at least 25 grams of fiber per day.

■ **STOP DRINKING CALORIES.** "This is one of the easiest food behaviors to change," says Francine Kaufman, MD, head of the Center for Diabetes, Endocrinology, and Metabolism at Childrens Hospital Los Angeles and author of *Diabesity.* Unless it is sugar-free, any flavored, sweet drink—be it soda, fruit juice, iced tea, lemonade, wine coolers, and so on—will serve up a lot of empty calories, usually with sugar that you do not need. And studies show that even calorie-free diet sodas can lead to weight gain because they trick your body into thinking all sweet things contain no calories and therefore are okay to eat without restraint. "Instead, drink only water," Dr. Kaufman says. If you want to give it some zing, drop in a piece of lemon, lime, or orange.

■ **WATCH PORTION SIZES.** One of the simplest and most effective behaviors that can help with weight loss is getting a handle on portion sizes, says Dr. Kaufman. Here are some quick, reliable portion guidelines.

- ■ The tip of your thumb equals one serving of margarine or mayonnaise.

- ■ A handful of nuts equals 1 or 2 ounces, or one serving.

- ■ One cup of cereal is the size of your fist.

- ■ Three ounces of meat is the size of the palm of your hand.

- ■ One ounce of cheese is the size of your thumb.

■ **BEWARE OF THE BAD OFFICE INFLUENCE.** "A big danger for people trying to control or lose weight is what happens in their offices," Dr. Kaufman says. Most workplaces are not healthy environments—temptations such as morning doughnuts, vending machine chips, and community candy dishes seem to lurk around every corner. And in the middle of a workday, let's face it—a snack can be a welcome distraction. But it doesn't have to be a sugary, processed snack. "When everyone else is having all that junk, eat a piece of fruit that you brought in. If it's an apple, cut it into pieces so it will take a while to eat—whatever you have to do to drag it out," she says. Dr. Kaufman also warns about the comments people will make at work, such as "Are you trying to lose weight?" Simply say, "No, I am just trying to eat healthy."

■ **CALCULATE THE CALORIES YOU DIDN'T EAT.** "In the Diabetes Prevention Program, one thing they did for the holiday season was a contest where people recorded the calorie count of everything they decided *not* to eat," Dr. Goldstein says. "So of course people went to their relatives' houses and came back with these index cards saying 'I didn't have this apple pie, which is 600 calories,' etc." To try this yourself, record every food temptation you resist in a notebook or on index cards and then tally up the total calorie count—you may find it motivating to see how strong your willpower truly is.

"Work Out" Your Diabetes Risk

"When it comes to diabetes management, exercise is absolutely essential," says Dr. Felder. The exercise in the successful lifestyle intensive group of the Diabetes Prevention Program study included a total of 150 minutes of cardiovascular exercise per week, or 30 minutes 5 days per week.

Dr. Felder concurs. "Exercise is important for three reasons: One, you burn calories while you exercise; two, your basal metabolism increases even after you have exercised; and three, exercise decreases insulin resistance [and therefore improves blood sugar management]," he says. "We don't understand exactly how aerobic exercise works to lower insulin resistance, but we know it does."

Here are some tips on how to safely and effectively exercise to get diabetes—or your risk for the disease—under control.

■ **TAKE BABY STEPS TOWARD FITNESS.** If you have pre- or type 2 diabetes, the American Diabetes Association suggests you talk to your health care professional before you start an exercise program. "People who are physically inactive absolutely have to be evaluated by a health care provider, whether it is a primary health care provider or a cardiologist, before they get out there and start exercising," Dr. Thomas says. Once you get the green light, start with 10 to 15 minutes of walking 3 days a week, and build up slowly to the recommended 30 minutes at least 5 days a week.

■ **MOVE YOUR HIPS AND SHOULDERS.** "You have two muscle masses that are most capable of using oxygen and picking up glucose, and those are the largest muscle masses in your body—your shoulders and hips," Dr. Marcus says. "These muscle groups will pick up more glucose and therefore prevent it from going where you don't want it to go. Walking is an extremely good exercise because it uses your hip muscles, and swimming is great because you use both your arms and legs."

■ **PUMP IRON.** "Research has shown that a combination of resistance train-ing and aerobics is most effective for controlling glucose level," Dr. Vagnini says. "Resistance training is excellent for diabetes control because muscle improves insulin sensitivity." The ADA recommends you perform strength-training exercises several times a week, and Dr. Vagnini recommends that your sessions last 20 to 30 minutes. You don't have to go overboard to see results; a study recently presented at an American College of Sports Medicine meeting found that men who did one set while they were lifting weights had better fat loss (19 percent versus 10 percent) and equal strength gains (21 per-cent), compared with men who did three sets.

■ **WALK OFF DINNER.** "I tell people if they have a big dinner, they should walk for 30 minutes afterward," says Cheryl Marco, RD, CDE, a registered dieti-tian in the weight management program at Thomas Jefferson University in Philadelphia. "Exercise gets the doors of the cells open so sugar can get in." More specifically, exercise improves insulin receptor sensitivity and enhances the uptake of glucose by the muscles and the liver. This leaves less sugar floating around in the bloodstream, where it can wreak havoc.

■ **PARTY WHILE YOU EXERCISE.** This doesn't mean you should go jogging with a bottle of champagne in tow, but you should make exercise social and fun. "If you plan to exercise at a gym, you are much more likely to follow through if you sign up for a class—aerobics, yoga, or whatever—than if you go it alone," Dr. Barnard says. You're also much more likely to get to your class or out to the sidewalk—even if you don't feel like it—if someone is waiting for you.

■ **MAKE LIKE THE TORTOISE.** Remember who won the race. "It is the slow, steady, and consistent person who walks most days of the week who is going to benefit the most from exercise—the people who run marathons and do extreme exercise actually get less benefit," Dr. Marcus says.

Skipping Meals

- **WHAT'S WRONG:** I seldom eat on a regular schedule.

- **WHY IT MATTERS:** Delaying or skipping meals can wreak havoc on blood sugar levels and—ironically, perhaps—lead to weight gain.

- **THE GOOD NEWS:** Research suggests that eating regularly spaced meals has a helpful effect on insulin response and that eating breakfast in particular boosts the effectiveness of insulin, which lowers blood sugar levels.

IN LIFE, whether you are skipping work, skipping out early, or skipping town, "skipping" is rarely a good thing. And the same applies to meals. Although it may seem easy to shove meals aside in the midst of your busy life, neglecting to eat breakfast, lunch, or dinner when you have prediabetes or type 2 will not only leave you hungry, it can have a dangerous effect on your blood sugar levels, weight, and overall health.

Just how harmful missed meals can be depends on your individual degree of diabetes risk. "If you have prediabetes and you skip a meal now and then, it won't necessarily present a problem," says Fred Vagnini, MD, medical director of the Cardiovascular Wellness Centers of New York in New York City. If you skip meals regularly, however, you will consistently cause your blood sugar levels to drop. And if you have already been diagnosed with type 2 diabetes and take insulin or medications, erratic eating can be downright unsafe; if you fail to eat and then take insulin, you will be at risk for hypoglycemia (low blood sugar), Dr. Vagnini says.

Hit-and-miss meals may also send blood sugar levels soaring, placing them on a roller coaster. "If you skip a meal, you are just going to get really hungry and then overdo it the next time you eat," says Francine Kaufman, MD, head of the Center for Diabetes, Endocrinology, and Metabolism at Childrens Hospital Los Angeles and author of *Diabesity*. Eating a massive quantity in one sitting forces you to secrete a large amount of insulin, which may increase your appetite—you'll ride an insulin wave, come down, and then get hungry again, she says.

Big meals create these insulin spikes because they stress your pancreas. When you chow down on a lot at once, your pancreas can't keep up with the demand, and it takes 4 to 5 hours instead of the usual 2 to lower your blood sugar, says Linda Yerardi, RD, CDE, registered dietitian and certified diabetes educator at the Diabetes Center at Mercy Medical Center in Baltimore. "Because it is overtaxed, your pancreas puts out insulin more slowly than it should, which leads to high blood sugar," she says.

And if that weren't enough, skipping meals sets you up for weight gain, a major risk factor for both prediabetes and type 2 diabetes. Studies show that although fasting may let you lose weight initially, when you eat again, you'll go back to your baseline weight—or higher.

Eat Often and Eat Well

Regardless of where you are in terms of weight or diabetes risk, you must find an eating plan that includes regular meals and works for your individual body chemistry, culture, and lifestyle. "I have some patients who have high blood sugars in the morning, and some who have high blood sugars at night—it varies from person to person," says Donna Rice, RN, CDE, a past president of the American Association of Diabetes Educators. "In order to be successful, your meal plan must be personalized. That means finding a nutritionist or diabetes educator who will target your plan specifically to you." Here are some things you can do on your own to keep your body well fed so your blood sugar is well controlled.

■ **GRAZE THROUGH YOUR DAYS.** If you have already developed prediabetes or type 2 diabetes, you need to think outside the three-squares box. "Sitting down to three large meals like we do in Western cultures is not a very healthy thing, unless your meal choices are such that you are not overloading your body. That is usually not the case with most people in this fast-food culture," says Alan Marcus, MD, a physician in private practice in Laguna Hills, California, who specializes in diabetes management and endocrinology. It might be better for people with prediabetes or type 2 diabetes to spread their allotted calories over five or six smaller meals and snacks throughout the day so they feel satisfied and don't overeat, he says.

■ **BREAK YOUR FAST.** When it comes to eating a hearty breakfast, Mom was right. "There is some funny physiology in the morning where people tend to be a little more insulin resistant than at other times of the day," says Barry J. Goldstein, MD, PhD, director of the division of endocrinology, diabetes, and metabolic diseases at Jefferson Medical College of Thomas Jefferson University in Philadelphia—even nondiabetic people have slightly elevated insulin levels in the morning. So make sure you eat *something* in the a.m., he says. If you aren't a breakfast eater, sip a glass of fat-free milk or drinkable yogurt, or eat an apple, some string cheese, or a few whole grain crackers. Have another little snack 2 or 3 hours later—whatever works to help you maintain a healthy blood sugar level.

■ **RISE AND SHINE WITH SOME PROTEIN.** It's wise to eat some protein at breakfast because it won't cause the spike in blood sugar that carbohydrates will, Dr. Goldstein says. His suggestions: egg whites, Egg Beaters, or a lean breakfast meat such as Canadian bacon. "Egg whites are particularly great because they contain low calories and high protein, so they will keep your blood sugar steady," he says. If you can't give up breakfast cereal, Dr. Goldstein recommends steel-cut oatmeal, which gets digested slowly and therefore keeps blood sugar under control. It takes 45 minutes to cook, but it's worth it. "If you don't want to take the time in the morning, make a batch the night before, and then stick it in the microwave when you get up," he says.

■ **HIT THE CARB MARK.** Counting carbohydrates should be second nature if you have—or are at risk for—type 2 diabetes. "You should see a diabetes educator to figure out exactly how many carbohydrates are appropriate for you, but in general, if you are eating three average meals and two snacks per day, you should shoot for 45 to 60 grams of carbohydrates per meal and 15 to 30 grams per snack," Yerardi says. To tally your total, read labels. And for foods without labels, invest in a good nutritional information book or check out nutritional information online, such as on the comprehensive calorieking.com.

■ **ARM YOURSELF WITH FOOD.** If you have or are at risk for type 2 diabetes, you should always be prepared for an unexpected blood sugar plunge. "It's the low blood sugar attacks that will put you in the emergency room, not the peaks," says Edwidge Jourdain Thomas, DrNP, assistant professor of clinical nursing at Columbia University. "So always carry something in your purse or bag to eat and drink." The snacks listed below are good options for an emergency blood sugar boost. They're also great for munchies between meals to keep blood sugar steady.

■ Protein bars: The best bars have at least 15 grams of protein and no more than 30 grams of carbohydrates; they include Slim Fast, Balance, Zone, and Detour bars.

■ An orange: "Peel it and leave the white part under the skin on it; there is fiber in the white stuff, which will block some of the carbohydrates in the fruit," Rice says.

■ An apple: When it comes to diabetes, the adage about apples and doctors may be true. Eat an apple with its peel (for the fiber), and you'll be in even better shape.

■ Cherries: "Cherries are a great snack because they have a low glycemic index," Rice says. Bonus: They're also rich in anti-aging antioxidants.

- Melon: Cubed cantaloupe and honeydew make a fast and healthful snack; keep a bowl of melon in the fridge and munch on it throughout the day.

- Nuts: Their healthy fat keeps you satisfied, plus they supply good-for-you omega-3 fatty acids. In an Australian study of 35 adults with type 2 diabetes, 16 people ate an ounce of walnuts a day, and the remaining 19 tried to get a daily dose of omega-3s on their own. The walnut eaters got the target amount, while the others got less and ate more saturated fat.

- Stuffed celery: Celery may not have much taste by itself, but stuff it with some peanut butter or reduced-fat flavored cream cheese, and you get a healthful, satisfying snack.

- Whole grain crackers: For a fast, low-carb bite, spread whole grain crackers with reduced-fat cream cheese, peanut butter, or tuna.

- Air-popped popcorn: Skip the oil and salt, and popcorn makes a great low-carbohydrate snack. Top it with garlic salt, nutritional yeast, or mixed seasonings, and you won't even miss the butter.

Smoking

■ **WHAT'S WRONG:** I'm a smoker.

■ **WHY IT MATTERS:** Smokers have an increased risk of developing diabetes. If you already have diabetes, smoking raises your blood sugar levels, making the disease harder to control. And the combination of smoking and diabetes dramatically raises your risk of heart disease.

■ **THE GOOD NEWS:** Quitting is a choice you can make that will lower your risk of diabetes and many other health risks, according to a study published in the journal Diabetes Care.

NO DOUBT ABOUT IT, smoking is bad for your health. Most people are familiar with the connection between smoking and cancer. But people with diabetes who smoke are also three times as likely to die of heart disease as nonsmoking people with diabetes, according to the American Diabetes Association. As if that isn't enough to get people to quit, scientists recently found a direct link between smoking and diabetes.

People who smoke are more than twice as likely to develop type 2 diabetes as nonsmokers, even without other risk factors, according to the Insulin Resistance Atherosclerosis Study. The researchers looked at 906 men and women who didn't have diabetes at the beginning of the trial. After 5 years, 25 percent of the smokers had developed type 2 diabetes, compared with 14 percent of those who'd never smoked.

"Primarily, our analyses revealed that participants who were current smokers had more risk of developing diabetes in 5 years, compared with participants who never smoked, even after adjusting for several other factors that increase the risk for diabetes," says lead researcher Capri Foy, PhD, assistant professor at Wake Forest University Baptist Medical Center in Winston-Salem, North Carolina. Interestingly, out of 128 people who quit smoking during the trial, 37 had no significant increase in risk, compared with people who had never smoked.

This study sends an important message. "Many young women who smoke feel that it will help them control their weight, and they think smoking will prevent them from getting diseases associated with weight gain, such as diabetes," says Dr. Foy. But they couldn't be more wrong.

Future research may someday reveal common pathways through which smoking increases the risk of both diabetes and heart disease, says Dr. Foy, but lighting up may also affect diabetes in unique ways. For example, besides nicotine, cigarettes contain many other dangerous substances, including cadmium, which has been linked to increased risk of diabetes. Cigarettes also contain chemicals commonly found in rat poison, the insect poison DDT, arsenic, wood varnish, and nail polish remover.

Scientists don't yet have all the answers about smoking and heart disease, either. But they do know it can raise blood pressure and cholesterol and cut the amount of oxygen reaching your tissues, which not only ups your risk for heart attack and stroke, it can also lead to miscarriage. In men, smoking can lead to impotence. It damages and constricts blood vessels, which can worsen leg and foot ulcers and infections, common complications of diabetes. Smokers with diabetes are also more likely to suffer from retinopathy, nerve damage, and kidney disease, not to mention frequent colds, respiratory infections, and joint stiffness.

With all we know about how smoking destroys health, especially for people with diabetes, it's unfortunate that one out of five people with diabetes smokes, according to a survey published in the *Annals of Family Medicine*. The survey also found that smokers were more likely to get diabetes at a younger age. Smokers were 50 percent more likely to report being in fair or poor health and feeling depressed. They were less likely to get daily exercise; check their blood glucose more than once a week; or make regular appointments for foot, eye, or dental care or see a diabetes doctor. Smokers were also less likely to have a strong support system in place, which can make quitting even more difficult. Quitting smoking is essential, however, if you want to protect your health.

Kick-Butt Basics

If you're a light or occasional smoker, you could try quitting cold turkey or at least quickly. Nicotine is a powerfully addictive drug, however, so if you're a heavy smoker (more than 20 cigarettes a day), chances are you're hooked, both mentally and physically. You'll probably experience withdrawal symptoms, which may include restlessness, sweating, headaches, dizziness, diarrhea, constipation, insomnia, and fatigue. The second day after quitting is usually the worst, according to the American Diabetes Association. Symptoms will gradually subside over a couple of weeks.

If you have trouble quitting on your own, speak with your doctor about nicotine replacement therapy to reduce withdrawal symptoms. NRT options include nicotine patches, gum, or lozenges (available over the counter) or a nicotine inhaler or spray (available by prescription). These medicines can cause

SECONDHAND SMOKE, MAJOR EFFECTS

Actual smokers get a toxin dose 100 times greater than that delivered to passive smokers—but secondhand smoke's impact on the heart is far greater than you might think. The effects of passive smoking on the cardiovascular system are, on average, 80 to 90 percent as great as the effects of active smoking. In fact, there's growing evidence that the heart is extra sensitive to the toxins in secondhand smoke.

Passive smoking can increase the risk of heart disease in a number of interacting ways—damaging the endothelial cells that line the blood vessels, contributing to atherosclerosis, and increasing oxidative stress and inflammation. Even brief but multiple exposures to secondhand smoke can have cardiovascular effects nearly as great as long-term active smoking.

Exposure to tobacco smoke also appears to increase the risk of the metabolic syndrome among teens, especially overweight teens, according to a study published in the journal *Circulation*. Researchers asked 2,273 teens and their parents about their smoking habits. The teens also got physical exams and blood tests to find out if they had metabolic syndrome and if they had been exposed to tobacco smoke.

Only 1.2 percent of the unexposed teens had metabolic syndrome, compared with 5.4 percent of those exposed to secondhand smoke and 8.7 percent of the smokers. Even more dramatic: Among overweight teens or teens at risk for becoming heavy, metabolic syndrome was found in 5.6 percent of unexposed teens, 19.6 percent of teens exposed to secondhand smoke, and 23.6 percent of smokers.

side effects, however, including raising blood sugar levels in some people with diabetes, so work carefully with your doctor. And you shouldn't use NRT if you're pregnant.

Follow the instructions carefully, and avoid mixing cigarettes and NRT. Remember, you're trying to quit. Gradually use less and less medicine until you're ready to stop completely. For a nicotine-free alternative, a medication called bupropion hydrochloride is also available by prescription.

Although quitting may be a challenge, the rewards will be well worth the effort. Here are a few more strategies known to help.

■ **MAKE A LIST.** Write down all your reasons for quitting so you can review them for inspiration when you're tempted to light up. For starters, you'll get healthier, live longer, save money, smell fresher, and gain energy.

■ **DO A HABIT AUDIT.** Take a close look at your smoking habits. When and how often do you light up? What tempts you, comforts you, eggs you on? What will you miss most? Write down your biggest fears and concerns about quitting. Then make a new plan. For example, if you're concerned about not being able to relax without a cigarette, plan a few healthier stress relievers, such as meditation, a warm bath, or getting lost in a great novel. If you typically grab a smoke to feel energized, do a few invigorating stretches or listen to lively music. If smoking's a social habit for you, decide how you'll manage the urge when you're out with friends.

■ **SOLICIT SUPPORT.** Speak with your doctor about your plan to quit smoking. As your health improves, any medications you're taking, such as insulin or other drugs for diabetes, blood pressure, and cholesterol, may need to be tweaked. If you're worried about gaining weight, work with a dietitian to create a new exercise and eating program. Enlist any family members or friends you can count on to encourage you to stick to your plan.

■ **CONSIDER TAKING A CLASS.** If misery loves company, quitting as part of a group may hold some appeal. Many employers, insurance plans, and local hospitals sponsor instructional courses for quitters. Check your local directories for smokers' information and treatment centers.

■ **SET A QUIT DATE.** Once you have a plan, choose a date to get started, preferably one when you're free of other stressful events so you'll have the energy to focus on your goal. A good time to quit smoking may be during the first half of your menstrual cycle, according to a study published in the *Journal of Consulting and Clinical Psychology*. The researchers looked at women (average age: 38) who had smoked 20 cigarettes a day for 19 to 20 years and had already tried to quit three times. All of them attended group counseling sessions about smoking cessation.

Tobacco withdrawal symptoms were less severe for the 41 women who quit between days 1 and 14 of their menstrual cycles, compared with the 37 who quit between day 14 and the start of their next periods, says lead researcher Kenneth A. Perkins, PhD, professor of psychiatry at the University of Pittsburgh School of Medicine. "Quitting produces withdrawal symptoms that are often similar to premenstrual symptoms," Dr. Perkins explains. "Giving up smoking during the luteal phase—the second half of the menstrual cycle—would have additive effects that could make the experience more difficult."

■ **RESIST TEMPTATION.** For the first few days, avoid situations and events you know will tempt you to backslide. Steer clear of smoky hot spots like happy hour at the bar; head for the park or the gym instead. Take this opportunity to

BRING ON THE BROCCOLI

Munching on broccoli might undo some of the negative effects of smoke, be it from your own cigarette or someone else's. According to a study published in the *Lancet*, the substance that gives broccoli its bite—isothiocyanate (ITC)—blocks the enzymes that activate the cancer-causing agents in tobacco smoke. The 11-year study of 942 men (both smokers and nonsmokers) tracked the intake of cruciferous veggies such as broccoli and cauliflower by measuring ITC in the subjects' urine. Averaging just one cruciferous veggie a day cut lung cancer risk by 35 percent, compared with those who ate them less often.

try your hand at a new hobby. While you're at it, purge your home of cigarettes, ashtrays, and lighters. Then give your home, car, and work environment a spring cleaning to get rid of the telltale smell.

■ **BE GENTLE ON YOURSELF.** If you slip up—and most smokers do—don't beat yourself up. And don't compare yourself to others, because everyone's experience is different. For example, quitting is harder for people whose nicotine craving calms after their first morning smoke, according to a study at Yale School of Medicine. Simply take an honest look at the conditions that triggered the slip so you can avoid them next time. Then try, try again.

Stress

■ **WHAT'S WRONG:** I feel tense and anxious because of a personal or professional situation.

■ **WHY IT MATTERS:** Stress hormones can drive up blood sugar levels, and stress can interfere with your diabetes-control efforts.

■ **THE GOOD NEWS:** Research has linked stress-management training with small but significant improvements in long-term blood sugar control.

STRESS: It makes you shake your fist through the windshield at another driver. It makes you lose sleep. It makes you gnash your teeth.

And if you have diabetes, it makes you lose control of it.

"Anything that arouses people—especially negative arousal—is going to raise your blood sugar. Learning to focus on your body's reactions to environmental stimuli, and learning some simple techniques of putting a lid on those reactions, is going to have a significant benefit in terms of your long-term diabetes control," says Richard Surwit, PhD, the codirector of the Behavioral Endocrinology Clinic at Duke University Medical Center in Durham, North Carolina. One of his fields of research is the relationship of emotions with diabetes control.

When you're faced with a stressful situation, your body gets ready to confront it or flee from it . . . hence the term "fight or flight." This valuable defensive tool protected our ancestors from animal attacks, but it's not as necessary for modern stressors like family conflict and financial worries, and it's certainly not good for you if you have diabetes. Some of the physical changes that occur as your body primes for action include increased blood pressure, higher blood sugar, and reduced insulin production. The so-called stress hormones that are involved in the fight-or-flight reaction—including epinephrine and cortisol—can raise your blood pressure and encourage obesity, notes Dr. Surwit in his book *The Mind-Body Diabetes Revolution.*

The stress that can mess with your blood sugar control doesn't just come from daily life—it can also come from having a chronic health problem. A 2007 study published in the journal *Diabetic Medicine* found that people with type 2 diabetes often worried about developing serious complications in the future. Many felt anxious when they weren't managing their condition as well as they'd like; they were "constantly concerned" about eating, felt deprived regarding food, and worried about developing low blood sugar. Patients using insulin had more diabetes-related emotional distress, compared with people managing their diabetes with diet or oral medication.

In addition, people who are significantly affected by stress are more likely to develop depression, which can make your diabetes harder to control (see Depression on page 239). "Taking care of stress is an important component of maintaining good blood glucose control," says Dr. Surwit. "It's a simple thing to do—it doesn't require that you make an entire change in your lifestyle, and it's something that involves a few easy-to-learn techniques that have big payoffs if people apply them."

Two Stress-Busting Strategies

In one of his studies, mentioned at the beginning of this chapter, Dr. Surwit and colleagues divided adults with type 2 diabetes who weren't using insulin into two groups. Everyone received five sessions of diabetes education, but one group also learned stress-management principles. These included a progressive muscle relaxation and cognitive-behavioral techniques, which taught them how to recognize thoughts and behaviors involved in stressful situations so they could respond differently.

After a year of follow-up, the people who received stress-management training had a half-point lower A1C, which is a long-term measurement of blood sugar control. That may not seem too impressive, but research has found that each percentage-point reduction on the A1C test (the National Institutes of Health recommends you keep yours under 7 percent) is associated with a 21 percent lower risk of dying from diabetes.

Plus, progressive muscle relaxation and cognitive-behavioral techniques don't cost a thing, Dr. Surwit says. You don't have to learn them from a psychologist, inject them, or make a co-pay when you pick them up at the pharmacy. They're easy to master. As far as diabetes-management tools go, that makes them pretty appealing.

■ **PROGRESSIVE MUSCLE RELAXATION:** In his book, Dr. Surwit calls this the best technique for most people for inducing relaxation. PMR shuts off the fight-or-flight response, thus lowering your stress hormones and blood sugar. In addition, it will teach you how to recognize and relax chronically tightened muscles, which relieves tension.

Practice PMR for 30 minutes a day for 3 weeks, then start doing several dozen 30-second sessions during the day each time you become tense. As you're learning the technique, do it sitting in a chair, not lying down; otherwise, you're apt to fall asleep. Here's the process that Dr. Surwit recommends, which is featured in his book.

Focus on different body parts in the following progression. For each part, slowly flex the muscles and concentrate on what the tension feels like. Now think the word *relax* and slowly release the tension, really focusing on how your muscles feel. Take your time between each step, and carefully note the difference between the tight, then relaxed, muscles.

- ■ Feet—flex so toes pull back toward shins

- ■ Thighs—tense by pushing the back of your legs into the bottom of the chair

- Buttocks—flex by squeezing together; allow tensed muscles to lift you slightly in your chair

- Abdomen—tighten stomach, pulling navel inward

- Hands—tense by arching them back toward wrists

- Neck and shoulder muscles—raise shoulders upward, let head tilt forward

- Neck—bend head to right side, relax, then bend it left

- Forehead—raise eyebrows

- Eye muscles—close eyes tightly

- Cheeks—tighten muscles by smiling firmly

- Finally, picture yourself sitting outside in the sun. Visualize the details of the trees and grass around you. Breathe deeply and enjoy the calm and relaxation for a few moments.

If you need more assistance with this exercise, Dr. Surwit's Web site—richardsurwit.com—offers a CD in which a calm, soothing voice walks you through the process.

COGNITIVE-BEHAVIORAL THERAPY: The stress you feel isn't just about upsetting situations themselves—it's also about how you perceive them. If you and another person see the same rise in the road ahead of you, and he sees it as a molehill and you see it as a mountain, which one of you is going to get more tired climbing over it?

Cognitive-behavioral therapy is "basically training people to assess what's going on around them, to determine whether or not their cognitions are congruent with reality, and if not, to change them," Dr. Surwit says. If you didn't get the job you interviewed for, do you take it as a message that you're unqualified to ever get another job, so you're stuck where you are forever? If so, your perception of reality might be out of line and compounding your stress.

Similarly, this method teaches people "to look at their reaction to what's going on, to make sure the reaction is congruent with how they're assessing and appraising the situation," he says. Once you've processed a stressful event, does your response generate an unnecessarily large stress reaction in your body?

This type of therapy can also help treat depression. In a study from the late 1990s, 51 people with type 2 diabetes and major depression received either 10 weeks of cognitive-behavioral therapy and a diabetes education program or just the education program. Six months later, 70 percent of patients in the therapy group experienced remission from depression, compared with 33 percent in the other group. The therapy group's A1C levels were significantly better at 6 months, too.

Dr. Surwit recommends the following steps for practicing cognitive-behavioral therapy on your own, which he discusses in his book.

- Explore your moods. Think about positive or negative moods you've had in the past week. What single word best describes each one? What was going on around you before the mood started? Get out a notebook and pen, and explore every little detail that might have contributed to the mood's kickoff.

- Pay attention to your thoughts. Amid the constant chatter of thoughts that crop up in our minds come worries about catastrophe or negative thoughts about our abilities. These can spin out of control if you don't stop them. When negative thoughts arise, write them down in detail in your notebook. What was going on right when the thought occurred? What kind of mood were you in?

- See if your thoughts reflect an accurate view of reality. Are any of your notes examples of all-or-nothing thinking? In other words, if one blood sugar test is too high, do you conclude you're eventually going to go blind? Other types of dysfunctional thinking, according to Dr. Surwit, include mental filtering (you see only the negative things about the world, not the positive), mind reading (assuming negative things about other people and the future that you can't possibly know), catastrophizing (expecting the worst), and "should" thinking ("I should have done that differently").

■ Explore your beliefs. Down deep, how do you see yourself? How do you see others? How do you relate to the world around you? Some of your negative beliefs about yourself and others may not be realistic, and it's time to get rid of them.

■ Replace your negative, unrealistic beliefs with new, positive descriptions of yourself. Hold them to be true as firmly as you believed the old, unrealistic ones.

Beyond these two cornerstones of stress management, many other small lifestyle changes can help you cope with stress better. You'll find more suggestions in Adopt a Positive "Diatitude" on page 327.

Sweet Tooth

■ **WHAT'S WRONG:** I can't resist sweets!

■ **WHY IT MATTERS:** Sugary foods not only break down quickly, they also take the place of more nutritious foods in your diet.

■ **THE GOOD NEWS:** You can enjoy the occasional sweet without upsetting your blood sugar balance. The trick is to make room for it in your diet, and plan the rest of your food choices accordingly.

WHEN IT COMES TO DIABETES MANAGEMENT, a sweet tooth is not so charming. "I don't think there's a sweet tooth fairy; there's more likely a sweet tooth devil," says Alan Marcus, MD, a physician in private practice in Laguna Hills, California, who specializes in diabetes management and endocrinology.

Sure, sugar tastes heavenly, but a craving for confections isn't just about getting a hit of sweet flavor. Sugar also has a mild druglike effect. "The taste of sugar triggers the release of opiates within the brain; in turn, these opiates trigger the release of another natural chemical called dopamine, which is the key to the brain's pleasure centers," says Neal D. Barnard, MD, adjunct associate professor of medicine at George Washington University School of Medicine and Health Services and author of *Dr. Neal Barnard's Program for Reversing Diabetes*. "Drugs of abuse—heroin, cocaine, marijuana, tobacco, and alcohol—trigger dopamine release, and sugars appear to do the same." So sugar not only tastes good, it makes us feel good. No wonder we're drawn to sweets, especially during times of stress.

Sugar was long blamed for diabetes—both for causing the disease and making it worse—but research has revealed that when it comes to blood sugar control, sugar has a few partners in crime. Any simple carbohydrate will act like sugar once it is eaten, including some seemingly healthful foods. "Sugar cravings go beyond plain sugar itself; some people crave foods such as white bread or bagels, which turn to sugar rapidly and release sugar into the bloodstream," Dr. Barnard says.

As a result, a few years ago the American Diabetes Association said you can have some sugar as long as you adjust your diet for it. "The change in diabetes management over the past 10 years is that we do not restrict sugar; we account for it," says Linda Yerardi, RD, CDE, a registered dietitian and certified diabetes educator at the Diabetes Center at Mercy Medical Center in Baltimore. "So if people want to have cookies, cake, or pie on a special occasion like Thanksgiving, they can—they just have to modify their meal to accommodate the sweet. This means you must manage carbohydrates in whatever form they come in, whether it is sugar, rice, potatoes, bread, or fruit." If you are on medication or insulin, you need to regulate your medications to account for the sugar and other simple carbohydrates you eat. But overall, the idea that people with diabetes must shun sweets has dissolved like sugar in water.

That being said, however, all foods containing simple carbs shouldn't be lumped together. "You can get just as much sugar in an orange as you can in a cookie, so carbohydrate-wise, the two are equal. But nutritionally, the orange is definitely better," Yerardi says. So even though you can account for sugar, you certainly shouldn't substitute a healthful, balanced meal with a big piece of chocolate cake; doing so would rob you of important vitamins and minerals.

The other issue is self-control (or lack thereof). If your sweet tooth has a small appetite, feel free to feed it. "My mother, who died at age 90 weighing 90 pounds, had a piece of candy every day for the last 30 years of her life," says Francine Kaufman, MD, head of the Center for Diabetes, Endocrinology, and Metabolism at Childrens Hospital Los Angeles and author of *Diabesity*. "But it was only one piece, and it took her 2 hours to eat it." So if you're satisfied with a small daily treat and account for it in your eating and exercise plan, it's okay.

The problem is that many people can't stop at one piece. According to the USDA Economic Research Service, Americans eat an average of 31 teaspoons of sugar a day—at least 18.5 teaspoons more than the World Health Organization's suggested recommendation of 10 percent of total calories.

So if your sweet tooth is ravenous, you will simply have to set tight limits. "Ultimately, what people need to do to calm their cravings for sugar is somehow satisfy them in an appropriate manner," Dr. Marcus says. "And that means eating things that create a sense of fullness; using artificial sweeteners when appropriate; and eating healthy, well-balanced meals."

Within those general guidelines, there are some specific ways you can keep your sweet tooth—and therefore your diabetes or risk for the disease—at bay.

▪ **REIN IN THE POWER OF YOUR CRAVINGS.** Part of controlling a sweet tooth is recognizing its strength. Can you have a small sweet treat and stop there? "I have had patients who are fine if they can eat a Hershey's kiss after dinner—that satisfies their chocolate cravings," says Martha Funnell, RN, CDE, a clinical nurse specialist and codirector of the Behavioral, Clinical, and Health Systems Research Core at the University of Michigan Diabetes Research and Training Center. "For others, it just adds to the craving, and then they want to eat the whole bag." Controlled portions will force you to bring a sugar binge to a halt. Reach for a bite-size candy bar or a 100-calorie package of cookies, or count out 10 M&M's (that's 100 calories) and put the bag away.

▪ **SAVE SWEETS FOR DESSERT.** Research shows that it's best to eat sweets right after a meal, not as a snack. A study done at Columbia University's College of Physicians and Surgeons revealed that participants who were given a drink containing only sugar got hungrier sooner than those who chugged one with both sugar and protein. The study suggests that eating sugary snacks by themselves may stimulate hunger and lead to weight gain—a big risk factor for type 2 diabetes.

■ **TRICK YOUR SWEET TOOTH.** Although you may think you need brownies or ice cream to satisfy your craving, all you really need is something sweet—like fruit. Dubious? Researchers at Cornell University's Food and Brand Lab proved it. They found that people who love sweets eat more fruit during the day than people who prefer salty snacks. You'd be surprised at how easily you can trick your mind into thinking you're eating a delectable treat. Hankering for a strawberry sundae? Stir some artificial sweetener into plain vanilla yogurt and top it with fresh berries. "You'll get the sweet flavor you crave, but you'll also get protein from the yogurt and nutrients from the fruit—all in a lot fewer calories and carbohydrates," says Edwidge Jourdain Thomas, DrNP, assistant professor of clinical nursing at Columbia University. If yogurt just doesn't cut it for you, have a small serving of vanilla ice cream topped with berries. Or, if it's a cone you desire, stuff ¾ cup of cantaloupe chunks into a small wafer ice cream cone for the desired combo of sweetness and crunch.

■ **MAKE AN EVEN EXCHANGE.** In general, you're allotted about 45 to 60 grams of carbohydrates per meal, including sweets and starchy foods such as cereal, rice, bread, tortillas, juice, fruit, milk, corn, potatoes, and peas. "I like to relate carbohydrates to money," Yerardi says. "I tell my clients, 'You have 60 dollars (or grams) to spend at a meal, and you won't get any money back if you eat less—you use it or lose it,'" she says. Although you shouldn't do it at every meal, if you find yourself in the midst of a sugar craving at lunch, for example, you can swap in a few cookies by swapping out two slices of higher-carbohydrate bread. Suppose you're planning to have a turkey sandwich on two slices of French bread—that's 30 grams of carbohydrates. Instead, make the sandwich with whole grain bread, bringing it down to 15 grams. Add two chocolate cookies for an additional 15 grams, and you're back to 30 grams.

■ **SEEK OUT SWEET TOOTH ANGELS.** Some seemingly sinful treats can be savored without causing diabetes-control consequences. "Sugar-free Jell-O and sugar-free Popsicles have less than 5 grams of carbohydrates each, so they won't raise your blood sugar," Yerardi says. Another safe splurge: fat-free, sugar-free Fudgsicles; for only 40 calories, they'll satisfy your ice cream craving and serve up 40 grams of calcium to boot. Many sugar-free foods contain some fat and calories, however, so don't go nuts; you don't have license to eat them uncontrollably. Make sure you read labels and account for the calories and fat appropriately.

■ **DON'T GET FAKED OUT.** Diet sodas have long been considered a great alternative to the real thing, especially for people with diabetes. But it seems they may have fooled us. "A recent review paper looked at people who drank diet soda, and it showed that they gained weight—and it was clearly not from the calories in the soda," Dr. Marcus says. The study, which was conducted at the University of Texas Health Science Center School of Medicine, followed participants who drank diet soda for 7 to 8 years; it found that sugar-free sipping was associated with a higher rate of overweight and obesity. The researchers hypothesize that because diet sodas offer sweet taste without calories, they may trick the body into thinking that other sweet foods are also calorie free and therefore okay to eat with impunity. As an alternative to diet soda, go for sparkling water with a wedge of lemon, lime, or orange; unsweetened coffee or herbal iced tea; fat-free milk; or just plain water.

■ **DIVE INTO DARK CHOCOLATE.** Not only will it appease a hungry sweet tooth, "a 2-ounce serving of dark chocolate daily can reduce cardiovascular risk [which goes hand in hand with diabetes] by 21 percent," says Ralph Felder, MD, PhD, section chief for cardiovascular nutrition, cardiology fellowship program at Banner Good Samaritan Medical Center in Phoenix and author of the *Bonus Years Diet*. Dark chocolate contains a high level of antioxidants, which makes it great for raising "good" HDL cholesterol and lowering "bad" LDL. Dove Dark is one of the best brands out there because it's made with Cocoapro cocoa, a specially processed cocoa that contains flavonoids. For a healthful version of chocolate-covered strawberries, dip the tips of fresh berries in melted dark chocolate. You'll get fiber and folate from the fruit and a dose of antioxidants from the chocolate, all while indulging your sweet tooth. Just remember that because it contains up to 11 grams of fat per serving, dark chocolate should be eaten in moderation.

The Diabetes Lowdown

Although they have suffered some scrutiny, if you have a sweet tooth and also have prediabetes or type 2 diabetes, artificial sweeteners can be a loyal friend.

The American Diabetes Association classifies most low-calorie sweeteners as "free foods," meaning they have no calories and (with the exception of sugar alcohols) do not raise blood sugar levels. Because the FDA has approved the use of low-calorie sweeteners, the ADA has followed suit. Here's a breakdown of the different artificial sweeteners and their pros and cons.

Aspartame (NutraSweet, Equal): This artificial sweetener is used in sugar-free yogurts, diet sodas, and other products. Because high temperatures can reduce its sweetness, it's not the best choice for baking.

Saccharin (Sugar Twin, Sweet'N Low): Saccharin might seem to be the bad boy of the bunch because it has gotten the worst press; studies giving large quantities of it to rats revealed that it could cause cancer. But according to Eric Yan, MD, a physician nutrition specialist at Valens Medical in Irvine, California, years of further research have shown saccharin to be safe for people. It can be used to sweeten both hot and cold foods.

Sucralose (Splenda): Processed from real sugar, this substitute represents a breakthrough for low-carbohydrate and low-calorie sweetening. Marketed under the brand name Splenda, sucralose has been modified so it doesn't get absorbed by the body. It has no aftertaste, acts like sugar in recipes, and measures cup for cup like sugar.

Sugar alcohols: Used in desserts, candies, and sugar-free gum, sugar alcohols include isomalt, maltitol, mannitol, sorbitol, and xylitol. They provide about half the calories of sugar and other carbohydrates and don't raise blood sugar as much—but they should not be eaten without restraint. To figure out how many carbohydrates you should account for with sugar alcohols, subtract half of the sugar alcohol grams from the total carbohydrate grams. For example, if a sugar-free candy bar contains 15 grams of total carbohydrates and 6 grams of sugar alcohols, you would take 15 minus 3 (half of the 6 grams of sugar alcohols) to get a total of 12 grams.

■ **STOCK UP ON STEVIA.** If you prefer not to use artificial sweeteners, you have another option—the herb stevia. "Stevia is ground-up leaves of the stevia plant, and it can be used as a sugar substitute that won't cause weight gain or raise blood sugars," says Eric Yan, MD, a physician nutrition specialist at Valens Medical in Irvine, California. Stevia, which comes in both liquid and powder form and is available in most health food stores and large supermarkets, has strong sweetening power—$\frac{1}{8}$ teaspoon liquid stevia equals $\frac{1}{2}$ cup white sugar.

■ **SWAP JELLY FOR SPREADABLE FRUIT.** Jelly may bear a pretty picture of fruit on its label, but you might as well sprinkle pure sugar on your toast or bagel, because that's what you're getting. Instead, use spreadable fruit—it's made entirely from fruit, so it provides vitamins and no added sugar. You can also use spreadable fruit instead of sugar in some dessert recipes, such as for pies, compotes, and snack cakes.

■ **BUY IT BROWN.** Just as brown rice nutritionally trumps white, when it comes to carbohydrate content, brown sugar is a better choice than white. The combination of white sugar and molasses is lower in carbohydrates than straight white table sugar—15 grams lower for every $\frac{1}{4}$ cup, to be exact.

■ **GRAB SOME GURMAR.** An Ayurvedic herb called the destroyer of sugar, gurmar (Gymnema sylvestre) has been shown to help calm sugar cravings. Research suggests that gurmar, which is available in most health food stores, slows the absorption of sugar into the bloodstream and stops it from being converted into body fat. Follow the instructions on the product label for proper dosage.

Traveling

▓ **WHAT'S WRONG:** I practically live out of my suitcase.

▓ **WHY IT MATTERS:** Taking medications and eating on schedule can be a challenge when you're on the road, especially if you're changing time zones.

▓ **THE GOOD NEWS:** In a 2006 British study of 493 diabetes patients taking insulin who received advice at an outpatient clinic, 95 percent said they were happy with the suggestions related to traveling. If more people become better educated on how to manage diabetes on the road, fewer people might experience complications due to travel.

NO MATTER IF YOU'RE on your way to a business convention in New York City or en route to the Caribbean for a relaxing 2-week getaway, travel can be stressful, especially in these times of flight delays and long security lines. "The stress of traveling, waiting in airports, not eating for long periods of time, and not having the right foods available leads to a disaster; traveling can be very detrimental to diabetes management," says Fred Vagnini, MD, medical director of the Cardiovascular Wellness Centers of New York in New York City. "And stress can raise blood sugar, blood pressure, and weight." Also, when you travel, changing time zones disrupts your sleep patterns, and you do a lot of sitting in airports, planes, trains, or a car—a bad combination when it comes to diabetes control.

And there's proof of travel's ill effects on diabetes management: In the British study published in the *Journal of Travel Medicine* mentioned above, the 493 patients taking insulin who traveled by air were followed for 3 months, and about 10 percent of them experienced problems while traveling due to low blood sugar.

"During travel, the biggest fear is that your blood sugar will go too *low*; that happens when you go for long periods of time without eating, like when you are stuck on a runway for 6 hours," says Martha Funnell, MS, RN, CDE, clinical nurse specialist and co-director of the Behavioral Clinical and Health Systems Research Core at the University of Michigan Diabetes Research and Training Center. Both high and low blood sugar levels can be dangerous, however, so monitor yourself for both when you travel.

Educate yourself, too. The British researchers concluded that patient education may help reduce the incidence of travel-related problems in people with diabetes. "When people with prediabetes or type 2 diabetes plan to travel, they need to meet with their diabetes educator or nutritionist to talk about the best way to handle the situation," says Edwidge Jourdain Thomas, DrNP, assistant professor of clinical nursing at Columbia University. If you eat healthy foods and maintain your exercise routine on the road, not only will you help control diabetes, you will have more energy and be more alert so you can get the most out of your trip, be it for business or pleasure.

Of course, "maintain your routine" is easier said than done when you're far away from your own diabetes-friendly kitchen, workout equipment or walking route, and regular daily schedule. Here are some specific actions you can take to keep your diabetes under control on the road.

■ **GET ENOUGH SLEEP.** Business travel often lends itself to burning the candle at both ends, which can be detrimental to diabetes control. When you're sleep deprived, your brain gets fooled into thinking it isn't getting enough fuel, says Alan Marcus, MD, FACP, physician in private practice in Laguna Hills, California, who specializes in diabetes management and endocrinology. "Plus [because it is tired], your brain uses only glucose for energy—it doesn't use protein or fat. When you don't sleep, you gain weight because your brain actually sends signals telling you to eat more carbs," he says. "So the whole concept of comfort foods—which are actually high-carbohydrate foods—is based on the fact that carbohydrates really do cause your brain to feel better when you are not sleeping enough." To improve your sleep away from home and prevent carbohydrate cravings, avoid watching late-night TV, don't drink caffeine after noon, or take a warm bath or shower before you retire.

■ **. . . BUT NOT TOO MANY ZZZS.** When you're on vacation, you may be tempted to sleep half the day away; after all, the point is to relax. Turns out that's a bad idea. A Japanese study published recently in *Sleep Medicine* revealed that oversleeping messes with your blood sugar levels. The study, which was done at Yale University on 1,709 men, found that those who regularly got less than 6 hours of sleep had double the risk of diabetes; when they slept more than 8 hours, however, their risk *tripled*. More specifically, the study looked at the participants' hemoglobin A1C level—a marker for diabetes—in relation to sleep. "The study found that your hemoglobin A1C levels will be lower if you get the right amount of sleep versus too much or too little," says Eric Yan, MD, physician nutrition specialist at Valens Medical in Irvine, California. A U-shaped curve indicated that there is an ideal amount of sleep. So what is it? Researchers haven't pinpointed that yet, but it appears to be somewhere between 6 and 8 hours. In the meantime, aim for between 7 and 8 hours per night, the amount recommended by the National Sleep Foundation.

■ **PACK YOUR WALKING SHOES.** "Frequently, when my patients with type 2 diabetes travel to Europe or somewhere else on vacation, they say, 'Gee, I ate all this food and I didn't gain any weight,'" Dr. Marcus says. "The reason why: They walk everywhere. They don't drive their car to the entrance of the mall and then sit and eat in a food court; instead, they are out there in their sneakers walking through building tours and up and down hills, utilizing muscles, and burning up all the extra food they are taking in."

If you do splurge on new and different foods when you travel (which most of us do), make sure you hoof it from point to point whenever possible, rather than driving or hopping in a cab. If walking isn't an option or the weather isn't ideal, take advantage of the hotel fitness facilities or pool—do whatever you can to burn off those extra calories. The American Diabetes Association recommends that you get 30 minutes of moderate-intensity activity (such as brisk walking) at least 5 days a week. The point is, if you're eating more than usual while away from home, try to move more than usual, too. If that's not possible, at least do as much as you can. Even a 10-minute walk around the block or through the airport is better than nothing.

■ **PACK A PICNIC FOR THE PLANE.** Long flights force you to go for extended periods of time without eating, so pack some healthful snacks. Stock your carry-on with fruit, a small bag of nuts, or a peanut butter sandwich on whole grain bread, says Linda Yerardi, RD, CDE, registered dietitian and certified diabetes educator at the Diabetes Center at Mercy Medical Center in Baltimore. Bananas and oranges are particularly great for traveling because you don't have to worry about washing them, she adds. Other good snacks include trail mix, individual packages of crackers with cheese or peanut butter, carrot sticks, walnuts, almonds, and one of Yerardi's favorites: big, hard, sourdough pretzels. "They take a while to eat, and they only have 25 to 30 grams of carbohydrates," she says. "If you're already transporting insulin, you'll have a cooler with you, so you can also pack some perishable items like fresh fruits and vegetables or cheese."

■ **RESIST IN-FLIGHT FARE.** From the giant breakfast muffin to the bag of chips to the carbohydrate-packed processed burrito for dinner, airplane food is as bad for you as it tastes. Even the nutritional value of diabetes meals is debatable, says Funnell (though at least you'll be served sooner). But because the food is on a tray just inches away from you, it's tempting—especially if you're not carrying your own food from home. In that case, grab a fruit smoothie, some yogurt, or fruit at the airport before you board.

■ **FLY BY TYPICAL AIRPORT FOOD.** "Airport food is the epitome of fast food," says Yerardi. "It's hard to estimate the carbohydrates in airport foods, especially when you are in a rush." During long layovers, pull a snack from your own stash (see above). "You'll have more control over the content of the food and be able to better analyze how many carbohydrates you have had,

COMPLYING WITH
SECURITY REGULATIONS

Security restrictions for air travel have recently become even stricter, including limitations on carrying medication and medical equipment on board. "Ever since 9/11, security measures have gotten tighter, and sometimes the screeners will actually take lancets or needles away," says Eric Yan, MD, physician nutrition specialist at Valens Medical in Irvine, California. Patients who have to go through long flights without their medications can suffer complications, and this is particularly true of people with diabetes. "There are some reported cases of people having their needles taken away, going into diabetic ketoacidosis on the plane, and then ending up in the intensive care unit when they landed—not a good way to spend a trip," he says.

Luckily, if you have diabetes and require insulin or oral medications, you can get a doctor's note that will give you permission to carry the necessary supplies on the plane. "I tell my patients to let me know if they're going to travel, even if it is a domestic flight," Dr. Yan says. "I'll write a note so their medications and needles are not confiscated at the security gate." Also make sure that your medications are proplerly labeled—ideally, in the pharmacy packaging—and that any supplies, such as syringes and insulin pumps, are packed with the insulin.

Another recent issue: taking liquids on board. If you normally carry water or juice with you to stay hydrated when you fly, you'll have to buy these items after you get through security. Any liquid you have when you enter the security line will be taken away.

which is especially important if you are on medication," she says. If you have to grab something at the airport, scout out certain types of restaurants. "Go to the deli and order a turkey and cheese on wheat or a salad instead of hitting the burger or pizza place," she suggests. "Whatever you do, avoid the pretzel stand because soft pretzels are extremely high in carbs, and they usually have been brushed with butter and salt."

■ **TURN THE AIRPORT INTO A GYM.** If your plane is delayed, don't waste the extra time sitting and staring at your fellow frustrated passengers; instead, consider it found time for a workout. "Airports are big places, and you can use them to walk," Yerardi says. Walking will help reduce your blood sugar, which may have inched up along with your stress level, thanks to the delay. First check your blood sugar to confirm that it's not too low; you might need a snack more than a walk.

■ **STAY HYDRATED.** In and of itself, flying is dehydrating. Add a lack of water and a tendency to drink beverages with alcohol (dehydrating) or caffeine (a mild diuretic), and you can become downright dried out. To keep yourself full of H_2O, start drinking a lot of water the day before you travel and keep guzzling during your trip. Bring bottled water in your carry-on (with the new security rules, you'll have to buy it at the airport after going through security) or close at hand if you're driving, and avoid beverages that contain alcohol or caffeine.

■ **MAKE YOUR DESTINATION LIKE HOME.** "As soon as you arrive, find a grocery store and stock up on some fresh, healthful foods," says Cheryl Marco, RD, CDE, registered dietitian in the weight management program at Thomas Jefferson University in Philadelphia. "When you book your hotel room, request one with a refrigerator—that way, you will be able to store fresh fruits and vegetables." If you want to make yourself especially accountable for your health while traveling, Marco recommends stopping at a local discount store as soon as you get to your destination and buying an inexpensive scale. "If you get feedback about your weight, you will alter your food intake if you see yourself putting on pounds," she says.

■ **WRITE A FAST-FOOD CHEAT SHEET.** Car travel can be even worse for diabetes control than flying, due almost solely to drive-thrus. "People make the most eating mistakes when they don't have a plan," Yerardi says. "So before you leave for a road trip, go online to various fast-food restaurant sites and fill a little notebook with acceptable menu items." Most chains post all their nutritional information online, so you can check the carbohydrate, fat, and calorie content of foods to make sure they will fit into your plan. "If you have all the acceptable menu items already written down, you can pull up to the drive-thru and know exactly what to order. Most people order the same things repeatedly at fast-food restaurants, so if you reprogram yourself to order something you know is safe, fast food won't be a problem anymore," she says.

■ **PLAN FOR AN EMERGENCY.** "If you take insulin or certain medications to lower your blood sugar, you should always have glucose tablets on hand, especially when you travel, because you never know when you're going to get delayed," Yerardi says. "In addition, always pack your medications in your carry-on, so they are with you at all times."

■ **CARRY YOUR DIABETES METER.** If your blood sugars are off due to the change in schedule, diarrhea, or other traveling woes, you must adjust your medications accordingly. "Make sure you carry your meter wherever you go so you can monitor your blood sugar and make the right decisions regarding eating and medications when you travel," says Donna Rice, RN, CDE, immediate past president of the American Association of Diabetes Educators.

■ **DON'T LET YOUR INSULIN GET JET-LAGGED.** When you take insulin based on a structured eating plan, a change in time zones can confuse things. "The suggestion I give to my patients is that if they plan to go west with a time differential of about 7 hours, they should give themselves an extra dose of insulin because they will gain time," says Dr. Yan. "If they plan to go east 7 hours, I tell them to lower their insulin dose a bit to compensate."

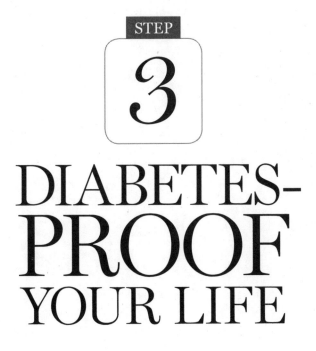

STEP

3

DIABETES-PROOF
YOUR LIFE

1. Know Your Risk

YOU'VE NO DOUBT HEARD the familiar Serenity Prayer that's so popular in 12-step groups: "God grant me the serenity to accept the things I cannot change, the courage to change the things I can, and the wisdom to know the difference."

That's a pretty good way to look at your risk of getting diabetes or suffering from its complications. There are risk factors you can change and others you can't; and with some courage and a lot of perseverance, changing the ones you can change may make all the difference.

It's also true—at least for type 2 diabetes—that the more risk factors you have, the more likely it is that you will get the disease. To put a positive spin on it: You have even more opportunity to address those issues and reduce your risk.

This chapter will give you an overview of diabetes risk factors, divided into the "can change" and "can't change" categories, which doctors would call "modifiable and nonmodifiable" risk factors. Keep in mind, though, that the dividing line between what's modifiable and what's not isn't always crystal clear. Researchers believe that some people are genetically predisposed to obesity, for example, while others are predisposed to high cholesterol. Still, even when risk factors are in the genes, you can do a lot to combat them.

Risk Factors You Can't Change

■ **AGE:** Type 1 diabetes is usually (but not always) diagnosed in children, teenagers, or young adults. Type 2 diabetes becomes increasingly common among people who are middle-aged or older, although, as mentioned in earlier chapters, its prevalence among younger people is growing. In a major national survey that tracked the number of new type 2 cases between 1988 and 1994, the average age at diagnosis was 52. Five years later, the same survey revealed that the age had dropped to 46.

■ **FAMILY, RACE, AND ETHNICITY:** You can inherit a greater risk of getting either type 1 or type 2 diabetes from your parents, but the influence has limits. Only about 10 percent of the people who get type 1 have a relative with the disease. Family history plays more of a role in type 2 diabetes, especially if your mother had gestational diabetes. Paradoxically, it's also true that there's more that you can do to lower your risk of getting type 2 diabetes, as we'll soon discuss.

Your racial and ethnic background can have a strong influence on your risk. Type 1 diabetes is more common among whites, while the opposite is true for type 2. African Americans, Mexican Americans, and Puerto Ricans are almost twice as likely to have diabetes as non-Hispanic whites. Prevalence rates among Native Americans, natives of Alaska, and some Pacific Islander groups are even higher.

Risk Factors You Can Change

Because type 1 diabetes is an autoimmune disease, whether or not you get it is pretty much out of your control (at least for now). Researchers are looking into the role environment plays in its development but haven't yet found definitive answers. On the other hand, modifiable risk factors have a lot to do with your risk of developing type 2 diabetes and the disease's impact on your body. In fact, researchers say that changes in lifestyle are your best protection against type 2 diabetes and can effectively limit complications of the disease, regardless of your racial or ethnic background.

Here's a look at the most important diabetes risk factors—those you *can* do something about.

■ **GENDER:** Nope, this isn't in this category by mistake—although you aren't likely to change your gender (and even if you did, your diabetes risk wouldn't change). The number of men and women who have the disease is essentially equal. The difference is being diagnosed: Significantly more men than women have diabetes and don't know it. Because diabetes can do a lot of damage before you realize you have it, and because there's a lot you can do to avoid that damage once you know you have it, being undiagnosed is a major risk factor—and being a man makes you more likely to go undiagnosed.

■ **HIGH BLOOD GLUCOSE LEVELS:** Having blood glucose levels that fall in the prediabetic range is probably the single best risk indicator. Studies have shown than 60 percent of people who develop diabetes qualified as prediabetic 5 years before they were diagnosed. For more information, see "Testing for Prediabetes" on page 19.

The American Diabetes Association defines a fasting blood glucose level below 100 mg/dL (milligrams per deciliter) as normal, between 100 and 125 mg/dL as prediabetic, and 126 mg/dL or higher as diabetes. Lowering higher-than-normal levels can substantially reduce your risks. One study showed that for every percentage point that a person dropped on a common blood glucose test, risk of diabetes complications fell by 40 percent.

■ **OBESITY:** This is another big one, if you'll excuse the pun. Obesity increases insulin resistance directly and indirectly throughout the body, which helps explain why 9 out of 10 people who are newly diagnosed with type 2 diabetes are overweight.

The good news is that you don't have to become as slim as a cover girl to substantially reduce your risk. A joint statement from the American Diabetes Association (ADA) and the American Heart Association (AHA) notes that losing just 7 percent of your body weight in a year, followed by lesser percentages after that, is "extremely effective" in reducing your risk of diabetes and its complications.

One way of telling if you need to lose weight is to figure out your body mass index, or BMI. A BMI of 25 or more is considered overweight and puts you at higher risk of diabetes. A BMI of 30 or more is considered obese.

Where you carry excess weight makes a difference, too. Having an apple shape, with a big roll of fat around the waist, is generally considered more of a risk than having a pear shape, with the extra pounds concentrated in your hips and thighs. However, a 2005 study by researchers at the University of Illinois and Harvard University found that overall obesity and abdominal obesity are both independent and valid predictors of type 2 diabetes—meaning either one raises your risk.

■ **SEDENTARY LIFESTYLE:** Yes, being physically active tends to go hand in hand with being heavy, but that's not the only reason it makes the list. (It works the other way, too: Being obese is still a risk factor for diabetes even if you're physically active.) Studies have shown that physical activity reduces the risk of type 2 diabetes by 30 percent in the general population. No matter what you weigh, exercise improves your body's ability to process blood glucose and reduces a host of other risk factors (including high blood pressure and cardio-vascular disease) that can promote diabetes or worsen its complications.

You don't have to qualify for the Olympic trials to reduce your risk of diabetes. Participants in the Diabetes Prevention Program trial were encouraged to engage in moderately intensive physical activity, such as brisk walking, for 150 minutes a week. That's a tad more than 20 minutes a day. Following that regimen and eating a healthy diet helped them lower their risk of developing type 2 diabetes by 58 percent, regardless of gender or ethnic background.

■ **THE METABOLIC SYNDROME:** Definitions vary as to exactly what conditions make up the metabolic syndrome, but most include high blood pressure, high levels of "bad" LDL cholesterol, high triglycerides, and low levels of "good" HDL cholesterol in addition to high blood glucose.

High blood pressure is especially dangerous and especially prevalent—as many as 70 percent of people with diabetes have high blood pressure. Diabetes weakens the tiny blood vessels that maintain healthy function in the eyes and the kidneys. High blood pressure can cause those weakened vessels to leak or burst, which can lead to blindness or kidney failure. One major study found that each 10 mm Hg (millimeters of mercury) decrease in mean systolic blood pressure reduced the risk of diabetes complications by 12 percent. The ADA recommends that patients with diabetes aim for a systolic blood pressure of less than 130 mm Hg and for a diastolic blood pressure of less than 80 mm Hg.

The ADA also recommends maintaining an LDL cholesterol level of less than 100 mg/dL, an HDL level greater than 60 mg/dL, and triglyceride levels of less than 150 mg/dL.

The above risk factors cover most of the major conditions that can help earn you a seat in your local diabetes treatment center. There are a few important runners-up as well.

■ **SMOKING:** Smoking exacerbates the circulation problems that lead to the most damaging complications of diabetes, plus it raises your risk for each condition that's part of the metabolic syndrome. How to address this risk factor? In a word: Quit.

■ **DIET:** A healthy diet helps reduce your risk of developing those same metabolic syndrome conditions, as well as helping you avoid obesity. According to the ADA, this means eating a wide variety of foods, including vegetables, whole gains, fruits, nonfat dairy products, beans, lean meats, poultry, and fish. The ADA also recommends choosing foods that are rich in vitamins, minerals, and fiber—generally, fresh foods rather than processed. With planning, however, you can still enjoy your favorite foods while you manage your blood glucose, blood pressure, and cholesterol.

■ **DEPRESSION:** Finding out that you have diabetes can be depressing. Dealing with it day in and day out isn't much fun, either. No wonder studies have shown that diabetes doubles the risk of depression. In fact, there's some preliminary evidence that depression might create hormonal changes in the body that could lead to diabetes, so there may be a circular effect involved.

Whether or not future studies confirm that connection, it's clear that people who are depressed are less likely to follow the good health habits that reduce their risk of diabetes or its complications. To successfully avoid or manage diabetes, sticking with a food and exercise program day in and day out can make all the difference. Depression makes that harder. If your low moods and negative thoughts seem to be more than a passing case of the blues, talk to your doctor. The better you feel emotionally, the better you are able to keep yourself in the best health possible.

2. Monitor Your Blood Sugar

IF YOU'RE LIKE MOST AMERICANS with diabetes, you think you're managing the disease just fine. In a 2005 national survey, 84 percent of Americans with type 2 diabetes said they had control of their blood sugar.

But many of them were wrong. The same year, the American Association of Clinical Endocrinologists released results of a study of 157,000 people with type 2 diabetes. The study found that two out of three people did *not* have control of their blood sugar, according to hemoglobin A1C tests that measure blood sugar levels over a 2- to 3-month period. In every state of the country, the blood sugar levels of most of the people studied were out of control.

And many are suffering the consequences. Nationally, experts estimate that three out of five people with diabetes have at least one related complication, such as heart disease, stroke, eye disease, kidney disease, or foot problems.

The good news is there's something you can do about it. Worldwide studies have found that when people get control of their blood sugar, whether they have type 1 or type 2 diabetes, they lower their risk of complications. Lowering your A1C test by 1 percentage point lowers your risk of eye, kidney, and nerve diseases by 40 percent, according to the American Diabetes Association.

That's why some doctors believe everyone with diabetes should test their blood sugar every day at home. Doing so, along with regular A1C testing, will help open your eyes to how well you're really managing the disease.

Monitoring your blood sugar is like crossing the street, says Gerald Bernstein, MD, director of the Gerald J. Friedman Diabetes Institute Diabetes Management Program at Beth Israel Hospital in New York City. "You don't cross the street with your eyes closed," he points out. "If you know your body doesn't handle glucose properly, you need to do the things that are necessary to get it normal."

How High Blood Sugar Wreaks Havoc

When glucose builds up in your blood, it's a toxin, says Francine R. Kaufman, MD, head of the Center for Diabetes, Endocrinology, and Metabolism at Childrens Hospital Los Angeles; and author of *Diabesity*. "In high concentrations, it builds up in certain parts of the cells, such as the lining cells of our blood vessels, our kidney and eye cells, and parts of the nerve cells," she says. The buildup leads to deterioration.

You won't feel the effects of high blood sugar until you experience a complication, such as nerve, eye, or kidney damage. "That's why it's important for people to know what their blood sugar is," Dr. Bernstein says. If you know when it's high, you can take action.

Diabetes is the leading cause of new cases of blindness among people ages 20 to 74, but research has shown that keeping blood sugar levels as close to normal as possible reduces damage to the eyes by 76 percent in people with type 1 diabetes; researchers say that may apply to people with type 2 as well.

In addition, diabetes is the leading cause of kidney failure, but keeping your blood glucose levels as normal as possible lowers kidney damage by up to 56 percent, research shows.

And controlling your blood sugar can help you avoid being part of the 60 to 70 percent of people with diabetes who have mild to severe forms of nerve damage, including pain or reduced sensation in the feet or hands, slow digestion, carpal tunnel syndrome, and other problems that can lead to amputations.

If that doesn't convince you to keep your blood sugar in check, think about this: If your blood sugar remains very high for a long time, it could lead to ketoacidosis, a condition in which your body metabolizes fat instead of sugar for energy. When your body breaks down fat, it produces ketones and your blood becomes more acidic than your body tissues. Symptoms include frequent urination, dehydration, and nausea. If it goes untreated, ketoacidosis can cause coma.

Make the Most of Monitoring

Because ignorance is not bliss when you have diabetes, many doctors say that anyone who has been diagnosed should begin self-monitoring. The more you know and use the information to manage your diabetes, the more you'll be stacking the deck in your favor, says Ann Albright, PhD, RD, director of the Division of Diabetes Translation for the Centers for Disease Control and Prevention in Atlanta.

Knowing how *your* body reacts is especially important because each person's response to foods and activity is unique. Two people may have completely different glucose responses after eating the same meal. And if you take insulin, testing your blood sugar is critical because the results will help you adjust your dose so you get just the right amount.

Perhaps the best advocates for self-monitoring are those who remember the days before home monitors were available. "I've lived with type 1 diabetes for 40 years, and I know what's it's like to not be able to monitor my blood sugar," Dr. Albright says. "It's like being in a dark place with a match and trying to find your way. Monitoring gives you the opportunity to have a brighter light and find the path to diabetes control."

Dr. Bernstein remembers treating patients during the 1960s before self-monitoring was available. "We didn't know anything," he says. "But once people started testing, we could alter their regimens, and they could take insulin exactly when they needed it." He has also seen the number of people who develop diabetes complications drop dramatically over the last 25 years.

Diabetes Rx

Living a long, healthy life free of diabetes complications means monitoring your blood sugar and taking action when needed. Here's how to make it a part of your life.

■ **FIND A FREE METER.** There's no need to pay the $30 to $60 a meter costs; diabetes centers and physicians often have coupons or rebates that allow you to get one for free. If your meter is more than 3 years old, manufacturers will usually send you an updated one gratis if you call their 800 number, says Ann Fittante, RD, a registered dietitian and certified diabetes educator at the Joslin Diabetes Center education affiliate at Swedish Medical Center in Seattle.

Once you get a meter, the most important thing is to learn how it works. Some require entering a code that comes with your test strips, Fittante says. And always clean your hands before testing. Hand lotion can cause you to get a higher test result, she says.

■ **CHECK YOUR INSURANCE COVERAGE.** Lancets can cost $10 to $15 for 100, while strips cost about $1 each—expenses that can add up quickly. The good news: Most insurance plans pay for supplies but require a co-pay. Remember to ask your physician for a prescription so your pharmacy can bill your insurance company.

If you think buying supplies is too expensive, even with insurance coverage, consider this: Having a diabetes complication triples your health care costs, compared with someone without diabetes.

■ **TESTING 1, 2, 3, 4—OR MORE.** People with type 1 diabetes should test their blood sugar at least four times a day—some test as many as eight times—to adjust their insulin for the best control, Fittante says. If you have type 2 diabetes, you should test at least twice a day, more often if you've just been diagnosed or if your blood sugar levels aren't under control.

If you're worried about checking your blood sugar away from home, don't be. Because the meters are small and give you results in a matter of seconds, you can discreetly do a check almost anywhere. Dr. Albright has checked her

New Testing Technologies

If you're taking insulin, you know high blood sugar isn't your only worry. You're more likely to experience hypoglycemia, or very low blood sugar, if you take more insulin than you need. When that happens, you may feel shaky, dizzy, hungry, moody, or confused or begin to sweat, develop a headache, grow pale, become clumsy or jerky, experience a seizure, or feel a tingling around your mouth. Someone with hypoglycemia should take three glucose tablets, a half cup of fruit juice, or five or six pieces of hard candy to raise their blood glucose.

Checking your blood sugar several times a day will help you avoid low blood sugar, but some people may still experience dangerous drops. That's why researchers came up with a continuous glucose sensor, a device in which a needle is inserted into the skin and a sensor measures glucose levels continuously throughout the day and sends the data to a handheld receiver.

In a study of 86 people with type 1 or 2 diabetes who took insulin, wearing the sensor and reading the results helped them gain better control of their blood sugar levels. Those who had high A1C levels at the start of the study particularly benefited from the all-day feedback. The advantage is that you see patterns in your blood sugar fluctuations, says Ann Albright, PhD, RD, director of the Division of Diabetes Translation for the Centers for Disease Control and Prevention in Atlanta.

"They're not for everybody," says Dr. Albright, because the sensors give you a lot of information every 2 to 3 minutes, which can be overwhelming. Still, sensors can benefit you if you have hypoglycemia unawareness and don't feel symptoms of very low blood sugar. Or they may help you improve what you're already doing. "Some people have good glucose control but want to fine-tune it," she says.

Sensors don't replace meters. You still need to test your blood sugar throughout the day. And whenever your sensor tells you that your blood sugar is high or low, confirm the reading with your meter before making a treatment decision, Dr. Albright says. Sensors aren't meant to be used constantly but only for 3 or 4 days at a time. They're usually not covered by insurance.

blood sugar in elevators and taxis, during meetings, and even before giving lectures in a large auditorium. Meters come with a carrying case, so they're easy to bring with you when you're on the go.

■ **SKIP AROUND THE CLOCK.** It's a good idea to know your blood sugar at different times of the day, so alternate the times you test every day, Fittante says. If you test only in the morning and after lunch, you may not know that your blood sugar rises dangerously a couple of hours after dinner. Aim for blood sugar levels within these ranges.

- 90 to 130 mg/dL (milligrams per deciliter) before meals

- less than 180 mg/dL 1 hour after a meal

- less than 160 mg/dL 2 hours after a meal

- less than 140 mg/dL 3 hours after a meal

Keep in mind that checking your blood sugar too soon after eating will give you a high reading. If you eat an apple and test 15 minutes later, you may get a reading of 180 or 190 mg/dL, Fittante says. For more accurate results, it's better to wait an hour or two.

■ **KEEP A LOG.** Your meter may have a memory that saves 200 to 300 readings, but it's a good idea to record your results in a log book or on a piece of paper so you can evaluate how you're doing over time. Some meters include software that allows you to download your results and graph the changes in your blood sugar. Don't forget to show your log to your doctor so he or she can make any medication changes that are necessary.

■ **LOOK FOR PATTERNS.** Monitoring is really about finding patterns, so it's a mistake to react to every isolated spike, Dr. Albright says. Instead, take note if your blood sugar goes up every time you eat a particular meal or consistently rises at the same time every day.

■ **MAKE CHANGES WHEN NECESSARY.** Monitoring your blood sugar is not only about poking your finger and getting a test result. "You have to do something with that information," Dr. Albright says. If your blood sugar is consistently within the normal level, note what you ate or whether or not you exercised so you can continue the habits that create good results. If your blood sugar is high after certain meals, figure out what you can do next time to see an improvement, such as eating less carbohydrate or taking a walk after lunch or dinner. A high level first thing in the morning may mean that you ate too much too late the night before, Fittante says, while low midmorning levels could suggest that your medication is too high or you're not eating enough for breakfast. If you've tried adjusting your diet and exercise to no avail, talk to your doctor about changing the dose of your medication.

■ **USE EXERCISE FOR BLOOD SUGAR CONTROL.** If you have type 2 diabetes, research shows that just one workout can lower your blood sugar and keep it down for several hours afterward. In a study of seven sedentary men with metabolic syndrome (a cluster of symptoms that include high blood pressure, high cholesterol, high blood sugar, and belly fat), researchers found that exercising after breakfast lowered the postmeal rise in blood sugar. The men who exercised before breakfast tended to burn fat.

Experts say that consistent exercise can improve your body's long-term reaction to insulin. If you're skeptical about how much exercise can really help, Fittante suggests testing your blood sugar before and after a workout. You may be surprised to see it drop 50 to 100 points or more.

Keep in mind that the effects vary according to the type of exercise and how long you do it. "If you ski all day long, your blood sugar may be lower for the next 24 to 48 hours," Fittante says.

■ **ACCEPT HELP.** The day-to-day management of diabetes falls on you, but physicians and diabetes experts are there to guide you, so enlist as much help as you can. In one study of 143 people in Brazil with type 2 diabetes who weren't taking insulin, researchers found that those who met with a nurse for half an hour three or four times a year for guidance on diet and exercise were more likely to have A1C levels within the recommended range of 7 percent or less.

In another study of 547 South Koreans hospitalized for diabetes, half participated in an intensive diabetes education program that lasted 6 hours a day for 5 days, during which they learned how to monitor and control their blood sugar, among other things. The other half received only brief information about the same subjects. After 4 years, the people who went to the intensive program had better control of their blood sugar and were less likely to be rehospitalized.

Medicare offers self-monitoring training for people with diabetes, Dr. Albright says, and the ADA is trying to get states to require private health insurers to cover training programs. In many states they're already covered, so check with your insurance company. Diabetes educators can meet with you one-on-one to assess what you're doing and give you advice about how to better manage your diabetes, Fittante says. Or you can take classes or attend seminars to learn more about controlling your blood sugar.

■ **FORGIVE YOUR MISTAKES.** It's easy to blame yourself if your blood sugar goes up, Dr. Albright says. She has heard people say they're bad for having poor blood sugar control. "You're not bad if your blood sugar is bad," she says. "You're struggling with managing a complex disease." Remember that when you start monitoring, your numbers may not be perfect; the point is to use them to figure out how to improve and take control of your diabetes.

■ **FOLLOW UP WITH REGULAR A1C TESTS.** Daily checks give you a snapshot of your blood sugar at one moment in time, but it's important to also follow up with regular A1C tests two to four times a year to learn how well you're doing over time.

3. Get Regular Screenings

AT FIRST GLANCE, diabetes isn't a pretty picture: It can make a real mess of your health. But here's the good news: Even though diabetes-related health problems are numerous enough to come at you like a herd of buffalo, you can see them from a long way off. And your doctor's office is a great place to spot them.

"If there's a silver lining in the cloud of diabetes, it's that many of the complications are slow and predictable, like eye disease, kidney disease, and neuropathy. If you see the earliest signs, frequently they are reversible," says Michael Fowler, MD, a diabetes specialist at Vanderbilt University in Nashville. "They happen in an orderly progression most of the time; and if you see complications beginning to develop, usually you can stop them in their tracks. If you don't have frequent visits to watch that sort of thing, that's when you worry about irreversible injury occurring before you can get it stopped."

Diabetes organizations recommend that you use the services of a health care team and visit these medical pros regularly. This team may include a primary care doctor, such as a family practice doctor or endocrinologist, for general checkups; an eye doctor; and a foot doctor.

Here's an overview of what to expect while visiting each of these doctors for regular checkups.

The Trip to Your Primary Doctor

According to the American Diabetes Association (ADA), how often you visit your doctor depends on how well your diabetes is controlled. If you use insulin or have trouble managing your blood sugar, see your doctor at least four times a year. If you're having complications or starting a new medication, you may need more frequent care. If those issues don't apply to you, schedule checkups two to four times a year.

When you go to the doctor's office, bring your glucose meter, Dr. Fowler suggests. Your doctor will probably study the records on your meter to look for patterns in your blood sugar—key information for determining if your medications need adjusting. Many diabetes specialists can download the data to an office computer for easy reviewing. If you know what's behind especially high or unusual blood sugar readings—maybe you ate a lot of cake at a wedding one day, or you had the flu one week—let your doctor know, Dr. Fowler says.

These visits to your primary care doctor also give you an opportunity to have blood, urine, and other tests to assess the health of your heart, kidneys, and other internal systems. Here's what you can expect your doc to check.

■ **A1C:** As you may remember from earlier in the book, this test shows the average amount of glucose in your blood over the past 2 to 3 months. This gives your doctor a better long-term sense of your long-term control than by just looking at the latest ups and downs from your glucose meter. Ideally, your A1C should be below 7 percent, which corresponds to an average blood glucose of 170. A lower A1C means a lower risk of complications. Dr. Fowler does this test at every visit (unless he's seen the patient within 3 months). The National Institutes of Health recommends it at least once a year.

■ **BLOOD PRESSURE:** You know the drill—stick out your arm and let your doctor or nurse check your blood pressure with the familiar inflatable cuff. This should be done at every visit; ideally, your number will be below 130/80 mm Hg (millimeters of mercury).

■ **CHOLESTEROL:** Your doctor should check your blood fat levels at least

WHEREVER YOU GO, REMEMBER YOUR A1C

As you go about your routine checkups, a lot of people will ask you for your number . . . your A1C number.

The result of the A1C gives you and your doctors a sense of how well you've controlled your blood sugar for the past few months. Even doctors who are chiefly concerned with particular body parts—such as your eyes or your feet—probably will want to know this number. It helps them assess your risk of complications and gives them a sense of how well informed you are about managing your diabetes.

The next time your doctor gives you your A1C result, memorize it (hopefully, it'll be a single digit!), or write it down and bring it with you on all your other medical appointments. It's a good idea to know the results from the past few A1C tests, for that matter, for an even longer view of your blood sugar control.

once a year. Keeping them in a normal range will help reduce your risk of heart disease and stroke. Your total cholesterol should be under 200, "bad" LDL cholesterol should be below 100, "good" HDL cholesterol should be above 40 if you're a man or 50 if you're a woman, and triglycerides should be below 150.

■ **KIDNEY FUNCTION:** When your kidneys are damaged, they may allow proteins that normally would stay in your body to escape in your urine. Once a year, your doctor should test your urine for protein, as well as measure the creatinine in your blood—a high level means your kidneys aren't working properly.

■ **FOOT CHECK:** A doctor should check your feet at least annually to ensure they have good circulation and nerve function; you may get your foot care from regular checkups with a podiatrist (see page 302).

■ **VACCINATIONS:** Ask your doctor about getting flu and pneumonia shots to reduce your risk of catching these illnesses; the NIH recommends that you get vaccinated each year.

The Trip to Your Foot Doctor

Many of us give our feet short shrift, despite the important job they perform. They support your body weight for thousands of steps each day and may spend much of their time crammed into sweaty, stinky shoes. They also can develop blisters and other injuries, which in people with diabetes can grow into medical emergencies.

When you visit a podiatrist, though, your feet will get plenty of attention. The regularity of your trips to the foot doctor should be based on how healthy your feet are, says Kathya Zinszer, DPM, associate professor of podiatric medicine at Temple University in Philadelphia. If you have no nerve damage and are at low risk for foot complications, annual checkups are probably okay. If you have nerve damage or other problems, you may need to visit every 3 to 6 months or more.

When you visit the podiatrist—also called a podiatric physician—the doctor will want to get a sense of your overall health, Dr. Zinszer says. Knowing how well your blood sugar is controlled and what diabetes-related problems you're having will help the doctor assess your risk of foot complications.

To ensure that your feet have enough blood circulation and the nerves leading to them are working properly, the doctor will feel each foot to note how strongly blood is pulsing through the arteries. He or she will also prod your feet at different spots with a thin filament—a plastic strand—to see if you can feel pressure. If it tickles a little, that's a good sign: You have sensation in your feet. The doctor may also tap a tuning fork and hold it against your foot to see if you can feel the vibration, Dr. Zinszer says.

To find more clues of impending trouble, the doctor will also check the skin of your feet. The color and skin quality indicate how much blood flow they're getting. If your grooming habits include shaving the little hairs on your toes, keep the razor away for a few weeks before your visit—your doctor will want to see if you have hair on your toe-knuckles, which is a sign of good blood flow. The doctor will also inspect your toenails for fungus, which people with diabetes are more likely to develop.

The foot doctor may also order an x-ray, Dr. Zinszer says. People with diabetic nerve damage in their feet are prone to Charcot foot, a condition in which the bones of the feet shift, giving the foot a distinctive shape.

The Trip to the Eye Doctor

As you know, diabetes can trigger a variety of health problems from your head to your toes. In the eyes, the disease can cause many different problems, which involve different symptoms and require different treatments.

Diabetes is the number one cause of blindness in adults from their 20s to their mid-60s, says Carlos Rosende, MD, chair of the department of ophthalmology at the University of Texas Health Science Center in San Antonio. With regular checkups, your eye doctor can track changes in your eyes and offer solutions that treat or slow the progression of any diabetes-related diseases. "It's very tough when someone comes in and they're in their mid or late 40s, and they're about to go blind because they really have never taken care of themselves," he says.

The most common eye complication is diabetic retinopathy. Your retina is a layer of tissue lining the back of the inside of the eye, and it contains a rich supply of tiny blood vessels. Diabetes can cause these vessels to leak fluid into surrounding tissue, causing blurry vision, Dr. Rosende says. The vessels also become more fragile, leading to rupture. You wind up with areas in the retina with no blood vessels, so your body grows new ones. These new vessels are abnormal and even more likely to rupture. The resulting scar tissue can cause the retina to separate from the inside of your eye, which is a serious and hard-to-repair form of vision loss. People with diabetes are also more likely to form cataracts. These commonly occur in the general population with age, but people with diabetes tend to get them earlier. Cataracts cloud the lenses, which are the "windows" at the front of your eyes that focus entering light so you can enjoy sharp vision.

Another more common diabetes-related problem is glaucoma, which damages the optic nerve that carries images from your eye to your brain. Excessive pressure within your eye can raise your risk of glaucoma, but you can also develop it without high pressure.

The problems don't stop there, Dr. Rosende says. The muscles that move your eyes as you look around can become temporarily paralyzed, causing double vision. You're also more likely to develop infections on the surface of your eye.

The ADA recommends that people with diabetes see an eye doctor at least once a year. If the doctor finds a serious condition that requires monitoring, you may need to visit more frequently, Dr. Rosende says.

Expect the exam to take about an hour. The visit to inspect your eyes for diabetic damage is far more thorough than a routine eye exam, Dr. Rosende says. You'll probably be given numbing eye drops to reduce discomfort and other eye drops to dilate your pupil—the black spot at the front of your eye—so the doctor gets a better view into the interior of your eye. The exam will likely include the following procedures.

■ **VISUAL ACUITY TEST:** You know this as the eye test with the big letter E. As you identify smaller and smaller letters on a chart, the doctor can determine the sharpness of your vision—a "vital sign" your eye doctor is particularly concerned about. At this point, you might be told you need glasses or a new prescription for them.

■ **EXTERNAL EXAM:** The doctor will examine your eyelids and the surface of your eyeballs, make sure your pupils respond properly to light, and check that your eyes move in sync.

■ **PERIPHERAL VISION CHECK:** To judge how well you can see at the edges of your vision, the doctor may have you cover one eye, look at him or her, and say when you can see an object (such as the doctor's hand) enter your field of vision from the side.

■ **GLAUCOMA CHECK:** The doctor will gently touch a device called a tonometer against your eye to measure the pressure within.

■ **INTERNAL INSPECTION:** Using a slit-lamp—a device containing a microscope and a light source—the doctor will inspect your retina and optic nerve. As you place your chin on a chin rest, the doctor points the light into your eye and looks into it with the microscope, which points horizontally. This is why you got those dilating drops—so your doctor can get a better look. The doctor may photograph the inside of your eye or make a detailed drawing to track later changes.

If you have retinopathy already, the doctor may do a more advanced check of your retina to better detect abnormal or leaking vessels. This requires injecting you with a dye that glows under special lighting.

Diabetes Rx

Got your calendar handy? Here's a summary of the medical appointments you should set up to stay on top of your diabetes—and away from complications.

- Visit your primary care doctor for a checkup at least twice a year, and more often if you have diabetes complications or you need monitoring of your medications.

- Get an A1C blood test at least once a year.

- See your foot doctor at least once a year, and more often if you have diabetes complications or are at high risk for them.

- See your eye doctor for a thorough eye examination at least once a year.

- Visit your dentist for a cleaning and examination twice a year.

4. Follow Prescriptions to the Letter

TO PROTECT AGAINST DIABETES and its complications, you'll need to faithfully follow your doctors' advice. That means making a commitment to healthy eating, exercise, regular blood tests, and, often, medication. Individual needs will vary, but each part of your personal prescription puzzle plays an important role in supporting optimal blood sugar control and improving your big picture.

The payoffs aren't just somewhere out there in the future, though. Studies show that, beyond avoiding health complications that may occur over time, there's an immediate benefit: You'll feel great—now! Harvard University researchers followed nearly 700 people who took medication for type 2 diabetes. After 6 months, those with improved blood glucose levels said they had more energy and vitality, experienced less anxiety, enjoyed a better social life, made fewer visits to the doctor, and felt better about their overall health. "Improvements in quality of life were consistent, suggesting that there is a physiological connection between healthy blood sugar levels and feeling good," says lead researcher Donald C. Simonson, MD, associate professor of medicine at Harvard Medical School.

You'll reap similar feel-good benefits when you take measures to control your blood sugar in addition to medication, say the researchers. That means regularly reviewing and revising your diabetes-management strategies with an endocrinologist. Schedule visits with an ophthalmologist for eye examinations, a podiatrist for routine foot care, and a dietitian for meal planning advice. Consult a certified diabetes educator to learn more about day-to-day care, and consider meeting with a mental health counselor because having diabetes doubles your odds of depression.

The National Diabetes Education Program urges people with diabetes to control not only their blood glucose but also their blood pressure and cholesterol. If you don't, you may need to add a cardiologist to your team. Following that doctor's instructions for diet, exercise, and blood pressure and cholesterol screenings, and, if necessary, taking blood pressure or cholesterol medication will help you prevent two serious diabetes complications: heart attack and stroke. If you already have a heart condition or you participate in high-intensity sports, you may want to work with an exercise physiologist.

Make a point of getting to know the support staff at all your health practitioners' offices, too. The people who schedule appointments and field phone calls are equally valuable parts of your health care team.

Is your head spinning? It's true that diabetes care can require an enormous amount of appointments and advice and possible prescriptions, but each aspect is worth it: Following all those doctors' orders leads to better blood sugar control and a better quality of life. Here's what you need to know to stay on track.

Oral Medication

Although diet and exercise are always cornerstones of care, the day you're diagnosed with diabetes, you'll likely leave with a drug prescription too, per the 2006 guidelines by the American Diabetes Association and the European Association for the Study of Diabetes. That way you'll have the earliest and best possible chance at controlling your blood sugar so you can prevent long-term complications.

For people with type 1 diabetes, insulin shots are the only way to keep blood glucose levels down (see page 312). But if you have type 2 diabetes, you won't need extra insulin as long as your body makes enough. Diabetes is a progressive disease, however, so insulin may eventually become part of your prescription.

The various type 2 diabetes pills lower blood glucose levels in different ways. Your doctor may prescribe one or a combination of the following.

INSULIN-AUGMENTING AGENTS

■ Sulfonylureas stimulate the beta cells of your pancreas to secrete more insulin. For these medications to work, your pancreas must be able to make some insulin. Examples include glyburide (Micronase), glimepiride (Amaryl), and extended-release glipizide (Glucotrol XL).

STAY ON TRACK: These drugs can cause low blood glucose (hypoglycemia), so pay close attention to eating on schedule.

■ Meglitinides stimulate your pancreas to make more insulin but have a shorter onset of action and shorter half-life than the sulfonylureas. The drug in this class is repaglinide (Prandin).

STAY ON TRACK: These drugs can cause low blood glucose, but the risk is lower than with sulfonylureas. Make sure you eat on schedule.

■ D-Phenylalanine derivatives help the pancreas produce insulin sooner after a meal and release the insulin for a shorter time, compared with sulfonylureas. This helps lower your blood glucose after eating and is less likely to cause low blood sugar several hours afterward. Nateglinide (Starlix) is currently the only medicine in this relatively new category of diabetes pills.

STAY ON TRACK: If you experience mild cold- or flulike symptoms, dizziness, backache, and aching joints after taking Starlix, call your doctor; they could be side effects. Studies show low blood glucose levels are rare with this drug, but they do occur in 2.4 percent of people taking it. Again: Eat on schedule.

INSULIN-ASSISTING AGENTS

■ Alpha-glucosidase inhibitors slow the absorption of carbohydrates, preventing blood glucose levels from rising too much. They work by inhibiting a specific enzyme found in the small intestine that normally breaks down carbohydrates into sugars. Acarbose (Precose) and miglitol (Glyset) are the two drugs currently available in this class.

STAY ON TRACK: Because these drugs work in the gastrointestinal tract instead of the bloodstream, they can cause bloating and gas. If you have digestive problems and you're on these meds, tell your doctor. If you're working with a dietitian, ask for food strategies to help alleviate the problem.

INSULIN-SENSITIZING AGENTS

■ Biguanides help your liver respond better to insulin, decreasing the amount of sugar it releases. Other beneficial effects include a reduction in plasma triglyceride and "bad" LDL cholesterol levels. Metformin (Glucophage and Glucophage XR) is currently the only agent in this class available in the United States.

STAY ON TRACK: Both Glucophage and Glucophage XR labels contain a black box warning—a black-bordered caution of serious side effects—stating that they may cause lactic acidosis, the buildup of lactic acid in the body. If you have a kidney problem, make sure your doctor knows how well your kidneys are working before you begin taking this medication.

■ Thiazolidinediones work to overcome insulin resistance by making the body's cells more sensitive to insulin. Examples include Pioglitazone (Actos) and rosiglitazone (Avandia).

STAY ON TRACK: Medications in this group don't cause blood sugar to drop too low—unless you're taking other diabetes medications, too. Make sure you're testing your blood sugar regularly. Avandia now carries a black box warning because it was recently shown to raise the risk of heart attack in people who have heart disease. But if you're on this prescription, don't stop taking it without first talking with your doctor, says Mark N. Feinglos, MD, an endocrinologist specializing in patients with poorly controlled type 2 diabetes at Duke University Medical Center. The study numbers were small and their meaning unclear, he says. And for some people, the benefits may still outweigh the risks.

What If You Skip or Skimp on Pills?

Perhaps no surprise: If you don't take your diabetes medication—or you don't take it consistently—your blood sugar will go up. You may not notice the effects immediately, but out-of-control blood sugar can lead to significant short-term and long-term problems, says Dr. Feinglos. "If your blood sugar goes up for a day, your eyes and kidneys are certainly not going to stop working, but it can make you feel bad. You can get dehydrated, feel thirsty, and pass a lot of urine. You may get blurred vision because the shape of the lens changes when glucose shifts."

Missing a few diabetes meds doesn't have the kind of obvious effect that, for example, skipping blood pressure pills does, where your blood pressure shoots right up, says Dr. Feinglos. But don't be fooled. If you shortchange yourself, you'll pay down the road. "When your glucose is chronically high, you open yourself up to all the complications of diabetes," he says.

What If You Take Too Much?

Although more people get into trouble from not taking enough diabetes medication, taking too high a dose can lead to low blood sugar (hypoglycemia), in which blood sugar levels dip below 70 mg/dL (milligrams per deciliter). Hypoglycemia can occur suddenly. Early symptoms of low blood sugar levels include shakiness and sweating, dizziness, pounding heart, weakness, and hunger. If you think you might be taking too high a dose, check the label and speak with your doctor immediately.

Medications in Development

The hottest new class of drugs available right now is dipeptidyl peptidase-4 (DPP-4) inhibitors, and they work differently than other diabetes pills, says Mark N. Feinglos, MD, an endocrinlogist specializing in patients with poorly controlled type 2 diabetes at Duke University Medical Center. They prevent the breakdown of glucagon-like peptide-1 (GLP-1), a small protein made in the intestine that reduces elevated blood glucose levels. Because GLP-1 is a hormone, to get more, you'd have to inject it, says Dr. Feinglos. A better option: Preserve your own GLP-1. The enzyme that does that is DPP-4. "So if you take a DPP-4 inhibitor, your own GLP-1 hangs around longer and, as a result, improves your glucose when you need it," he explains.

DPP-4 inhibitors are glucose dependent, meaning they stimulate the release of insulin only when your blood glucose levels are elevated rather than all the time. DPP-4 inhibitors are less likely than some other diabetes drugs to cause weight gain, raise cholesterol levels, or cause hypoglycemia.

Sitagliptin (Januvia) was the first to gain FDA approval. Studies found it reduced A1C levels by an average of 0.6 percent in 18 weeks and 0.8 percent in 24 weeks in people with A1C levels of 8 percent. Sitagliptin can be taken alone or in combination with metformin or pioglitazone.

Other DPP-4 inhibitors in development include Vildagliptin (Galvus), which is in advanced-stage development pending FDA approval.

Insulin and Other Injectable Drugs

While not a cure, insulin is the most powerful glucose-lowering agent available. Insulin therapies administered two or more times per day through injections or other methods can help you stabilize and manage diabetes and delay or avoid complications.

Most people start taking oral drugs before moving on to insulin shots. But your doctor may prescribe injections in combination with pills, depending on your blood sugar levels, your overall health, and how long you've had diabetes.

Insulin comes in several types that work at varying speeds, from rapid-acting to very long-acting. Many people with insulin-dependent diabetes take two different types. How quickly or slowly insulin works in your body depends on your own response, your injection site, the type and amount of exercise you do, and the length of time between your shot and exercise. Your doctor may also prescribe synthetic forms of other hormones that work with insulin, as discussed below.

- Rapid-acting insulin starts working 5 to 15 minutes after you inject it, peaks in about 1 hour, and keeps working for 2 to 4 hours. Examples include insulin lispro (Humalog), insulin aspart (NovoLog), and insulin glulisine (Apidra).

  STAY ON TRACK: Check the package inserts for product-specific directions because they vary slightly between brands.

- Regular or short-acting insulin starts working about 30 minutes after you inject it, peaks in about 2 to 3 hours, and keeps working for 3 to 6 hours.

  STAY ON TRACK: The higher your dose, the longer the effects last. Plan your day and check your blood glucose ahead of time to help predict how much you'll need.

- Intermediate-acting insulin starts working 2 to 4 hours after you inject it, peaks in about 4 to 12 hours, and keeps working for 12 to 18 hours. NPH, the only intermediate-acting insulin currently marketed, is often used in combination with regular insulin.

  STAY ON TRACK: If you're mixing insulins, ask your doctor about using convenient prefilled pens.

- Long-acting insulin starts working 6 to 10 hours after injection and usually lasts for 20 to 24 hours. There are two long-acting insulin analogues (manmade forms of the hormone), glargine (Lantus) and detemir (Levimir) that tend to lower glucose levels fairly evenly over a 24-hour period, with less of a peak of action than ultralente (another long-acting synthetic insulin).

STAY ON TRACK: Because long-acting insulins don't provide enough of a peak to cover mealtime, you may need to inject rapid- or short-acting regular insulin before eating. The vials for all types are clear, so make sure you choose the correct one when you need it.

OTHER INJECTABLE MEDICATIONS

- Pramlintide (Symlin) is a synthetic form of the hormone amylin, which is produced along with insulin by the beta cells in the pancreas. Amylin, insulin, and glucagon work together to keep your blood sugar levels in balance. You inject Symlin at mealtime just like insulin. Other notable benefits: For most people, Symlin isn't likely to cause low blood sugar or weight gain and may even promote modest weight loss.

  STAY ON TRACK: Never mix Symlin and insulin in the same syringe because insulin can have a negative effect on Symlin. Even with careful planning, some people may experience low blood glucose levels about 3 hours after injecting Symlin. This reaction is most common in those with type 1 diabetes. Still it's smart to be prepared—make sure emergency snacks are always handy.

- Exenatide (Byetta) is a synthetic version of exendin-4, a hormone that lowers elevated blood glucose levels by increasing insulin secretion. Along with blood sugar control, you may experience modest weight loss and are less likely to experience low blood sugar.

  STAY ON TRACK: This drug, which you inject at mealtime, may initially cause nausea as a side effect. If this is severe or continues, speak with your doctor about changing your prescription.

Insulin Delivery Devices

Most people give themselves shots of insulin with a bottle and a syringe. However, researchers are exploring easier delivery methods, including patches, surgically implanted capsules, and inhaler devices. In fact, the FDA approved the first inhaled powder form of insulin, Exubera, in early 2006 for treating adults with type 1 or 2 diabetes, but Pfizer pulled it off the market in 2007 when the product failed to gain the acceptance of patients and physicians due to side effects.

It's doubtful that insulin will ever be developed as a pill because it is a protein; that means your body would break it down and digest it before it could get into your bloodstream. But insulin-delivery devices have become more convenient in recent years. Here are two to consider. (No matter what device you choose, make sure you learn to use it correctly.)

- Insulin pens can be helpful if you take at least three doses of insulin a day and want to carry insulin with you. The device looks like a pen with a cartridge that holds 150 or 300 units of insulin. Its tip contains a fine, short needle, similar to one on an insulin syringe. You simply turn a dial to select the desired dose and press a plunger to deliver the insulin just under the skin. The newest version, HumaPen Memoir, digitally records your time and dosage data. If you tend to forget these things, this can keep you on track and give you better blood sugar control.

- Insulin pumps, commonly used for type 1 diabetes, can also work for people with type 2 diabetes. Instead of taking a series of injections during the day, a pump delivers insulin as an infusion from a small plastic catheter inserted under the skin. The device is a little smaller than a cigarette pack and has a computerized system that delivers insulin gradually throughout the day, offering a lot of flexibility in delivery. Also, many studies show that the pump results in better blood sugar control and reduced rates of hypoglycemia, compared with multiple daily injections. The disadvantages: You're attached to this little device, and it may cause weight gain.

Diabetes Rx

Try these everyday strategies to make sure you follow your doctors' prescriptions to the letter.

■ **START WITH SAVVY SELF-CARE.** Follow your health care team's advice for daily meal planning, physical activity, and other lifestyle changes. "The important thing to remember is that part of your prescription is diet and exercise," says Dr. Feinglos. "The other parts of the prescription are not going to work if this one isn't working."

■ **CHART YOUR WELL-BEING.** Let's face it, sometimes your medication schedule can get lost in the shuffle of day-to-day life. In fact, research shows that only one-third of people with type 2 diabetes have their prescriptions filled often enough to take most of their meds. One way to stay on top of the disease is to keep a daily journal, recording when you take your meds as well as how you feel, physically and emotionally. This can help you stay focused and motivated to stick with the program. Even small downward shifts in blood glucose levels can result in improved well-being, says Dr. Simonson. After 4 to 8 weeks on medication, most people feel noticeably peppier. Your journal will offer written proof of your improvement.

■ **KEEP IN TOUCH WITH THE TEAM.** To make the best use of your health care team, make regular appointments and come prepared. Examine your feet carefully each day, and tell your podiatrist about any changes. Check your mouth for gum or tooth problems, and alert your dentist to any problems as soon as they occur. Keep your eyeglasses or contact lens prescription current, and get blood pressure screenings on schedule. And keep your endocrinologist up to speed on any and all changes.

■ **AVOID PRESCRIPTION DRUG ERRORS.** Work with your pharmacist to get on a midmonth refill cycle. Why then? Filling your prescription at the start of the month may be hazardous to your health, suggests a study from the University of California, San Diego. Researchers analyzed the cases of roughly 130,000 people who died from prescription errors and found that deaths were 25 percent more common the first week of the month than in subsequent weeks. Prescription drug purchases jump early each month, when Social Security and welfare checks go out, says study coauthor David Phillips, PhD. And pharmacists tend to make more errors—doling out the wrong drug or dose—when their workloads are heavier. Always double-check refills before you leave the pharmacy.

■ **CARRY A LIST OF YOUR MEDS.** Taking a number of drugs at the same time can lead to dangerous interactions or unpleasant side effects, or it can render one or more of the drugs ineffective. Keep a complete record in your wallet, listing each drug's name, dosage, prescribing doctor, and pharmacy. Also include any over-the-counter medications, vitamins, and herbs you're taking, and note any environmental and drug allergies you're aware of. Share this list with your health care team.

■ **WHEN IN DOUBT, CHECK IT OUT.** To avoid medication interactions, talk with your doctor before taking any medication, including vitamins, supplements, and OTCs. Menopausal hormone replacement therapy may pose a particular risk to women with diabetes, according to a 2002 report from the Women's Health Initiative. The HRT used in the study increased levels of triglycerides (fatlike cholesterol found in the bloodstream). This is a red flag for women with diabetes, who may already have higher triglyceride levels. If you currently use hormone therapy, talk with your doctor before stopping your medication.

■ **READ THE PACKAGE INSERTS.** When you get a new medication, whether prescription or OTC, read the information that comes with it. If you don't understand or can't read all that fine print, ask your doctor or pharmacist for an explanation.

■ **TEST BEST.** Ask your doctor which glucose monitor is best for you and how often to use it. Then verify your monitor's accuracy and your skill with it by taking it with you to your doctor's appointment. Run a test at the same time as a venous test; the doctor's results should come within 15 percent of your monitor's number. Track your readings in a log or diary.

■ **MONITOR YOUR MAIL.** If you order supplies by mail, make sure they arrive in good condition. For example, shipping during hot or icy weather can damage

The Diabetes Lowdown

You can cut your need for diabetes meds by upping your lifestyle quotient, experts say. "If you change your lifestyle habits by eating right, exercising more, or losing weight—which are things that make your own insulin work better—then you'll need fewer medications to help your insulin or replace it," says Mark N. Feinglos, MD, an endocrinologist specializing in patients with poorly controlled type 2 diabetes at Duke University Medical Center. Some people think they can just sit on the couch and stop trying once they're on diabetes meds. But in the absence of healthy lifestyle habits, no medication is going to work, he says.

Lifestyle changes are the important first line of defense. British researchers recently analyzed several well-controlled clinical studies comparing drugs with lifestyle changes in 8,084 people with prediabetes. They found that lifestyle changes, such as exercising and eating a healthier diet, work just as well as drug therapy to prevent or delay the progression to diabetes.

"The diet-and-exercise piece is really the cornerstone of what you're doing to treat your diabetes," says Dr. Feinglos. "Diabetes is basically a fuel distribution problem—the inability to handle a caloric load properly because your mechanisms for doing so are impaired. If you make a habit of delivering less fuel, it's easier for your body to transport it where it needs to go."

insulin. Ask your supplier how the bottles are kept during shipping—are they packed in iced or gel-packed insulated containers?— and check them carefully for broken seals, leaks, or discoloration before use.

■ **STORE YOUR MEDICATION SAFELY.** Check the labels for storage information and to see how long your insulin will last after opening. Store extra bottles in the refrigerator. For comfort, let the insulin warm up to room temperature before you inject it. Keeping insulin in the freezer or your car can damage the drug.

5. Trim Your Waistline

IF IT'S BEEN A WHILE since your last serious attempt to lose weight, you may be in for some surprises.

▓ **SURPRISE #1: IT'S NOT JUST HOW MUCH YOU WEIGH, IT'S WHERE YOUR WEIGHT IS.** The evidence couldn't be clearer: Being overweight is a leading risk factor for type 2 diabetes. But while you may obsess about the extra padding on your hips, thighs, and backside, to really diabetes-proof your body, zero in on your waistline. There's compelling evidence that fat concentrated around the abdomen, called visceral fat, is more of a threat than fat stored in the lower body. Further, some research suggests that it is waist circumference—which assesses abdominal fat in particular—that explains obesity-related health risk rather than body mass index (BMI), which estimates overall body fat.

Women whose waistlines are more than 35 inches and men with waists greater than 40 inches are in risky territory. Alarmingly, in the World Heart Federation's 2005 Shape of the Nations survey, only 40 percent of Americans associated a supersized waistline with increased risk for heart disease.

▓ **SURPRISE #2: YOU CAN LOOK SLIM ON THE OUTSIDE BUT BE FAT ON THE INSIDE.** Although 80 percent of people with type 2 diabetes are overweight, people with normal BMIs can store fat in their bellies, especially if they live less-than-healthy lifestyles. Even if you're relatively lean, if your waistline grows, so does your risk for heart disease and diabetes.

Further, waistlines tend to thicken with age, even if weight doesn't change. For example, in women age 35 and over, hormonal changes can alter the way the female body stores fat. That means your hips, legs, and arms get leaner, while your midsection expands.

But take heart. Dropping a small amount of weight—and nipping a few inches off your middle—can significantly benefit your health. Your keys to success: Think waist as well as weight, and make lifestyle changes you can live with.

BMI: Only Part of the Story

If you're like many people, you know your BMI as well as your social security number. Millions of Web sites allow you to plug in your height and weight, press "Calculate BMI," and learn instantly if your weight is putting your health at risk. A BMI of 25 or more suggests overweight, excess body fat, and increased risk for health problems.

But while BMI is a reliable assessment tool, it isn't foolproof. Among researchers, "BMI is becoming less popular because the correlation between BMI as a marker of body fatness varies by age, sex, and race," says Jason Lazar, MD, director of noninvasive cardiology and visiting associate professor of medicine at the SUNY Downstate Medical Center in Brooklyn.

Further, BMI doesn't distinguish between weight that comes from lean muscle mass and weight that's pure fat. That means BMI can overestimate body fat in ultrafit people, such as professional athletes or bodybuilders, and underestimate it in those who have lost muscle mass, such as many elderly people. And it's possible to have a BMI in the healthy range but still have an unhealthy amount of belly fat.

Recent findings suggest that waist circumference is a stronger marker of health risk. In one study, for example, researchers led by the Medical College of Wisconsin analyzed health data from 10,969 men and women who took part in the third National Health and Nutrition Examination Survey (NHANES III). They found that waist size correlated better than BMI with risk factors for heart disease, such as high blood pressure, elevated blood sugar, and high cholesterol.

Waist Circumference: Tale of the Tape

Waist circumference is a basic tool but a powerful one. "It has gotten to where we have almost put aside the scale for a tape measure," says Dr. Lazar.

In one study, researchers from Queen's University in Kingston, Ontario, Canada, analyzed both BMI and waist circumference in about 15,000 men and women who took part in NHANES III. The researchers found that for every 1-inch increase in men's waist circumference, blood pressure increased by 10 percent, total cholesterol rose by 8 percent, "good" HDL cholesterol declined by 15 percent, triglycerides climbed by 18 percent, and risk for metabolic syndrome increased by 18 percent. Women showed similar increases.

More compelling evidence that connects waist size to disease risk comes from the 2007 International Day for the Evaluation of Abdominal Obesity (IDEA), a study of 168,000 people in 63 countries. This study found that—compared with the quarter of participants with the slimmest waists—diabetes risk increased nearly sixfold for the quarter of women with the widest waists and threefold for the quarter of men with the biggest bellies.

The IDEA study also associated wide waists with heart disease. For women, each 6-inch increase over a waistline measurement of $31\frac{1}{2}$ inches equated to a 40 percent increase in risk. For men, each $5\frac{1}{2}$-inch increase over 37 inches increased the risk of heart disease by 35 percent. (The IDEA study used the International Diabetes Federation's criteria for abdominal obesity, which use smaller waist circumferences to assess risk.)

Why are apple-shaped folks, who carry their extra weight around their middles, more vulnerable to insulin resistance and heart disease than "pears," whose excess fat pads their lower bodies? In a word: inflammation. Visceral fat is more metabolically active than fat stored in the lower body.

"Visceral fat secretes hormones and other chemicals called cytokines, some of which start a process of inflammation in the body," says Osama Hamdy, MD, PhD, an obesity researcher at the Joslin Diabetes Center in Boston. This chronic inflammation causes systemwide damage, which makes the body more resistant to the action of insulin and speeds up atherosclerosis (hardening of the arteries) and heart disease.

Visceral fat also is linked to extra fat storage in the liver—which can raise blood sugar levels—and to extra fat in muscle cells, which makes them resist insulin. As a result, blood sugar can rise to dangerous levels.

Slim on the Outside, Fat Within

It's relatively easy to tell if you're packing extra pounds or need to minimize your middle. But what if you weigh about what you should, according to BMI calculations? You're fine, right?

Not so fast. While it's desirable to be at a healthy weight, "weight alone is not the issue," says Richard W. Nesto, MD, of the Lahey Clinic Medical Center in Burlington, Massachusetts. "There are plenty of people who are thin but insulin-resistant and people who are fat but insulin-sensitive."

Several studies have examined people classified as "metabolically obese but normal weight" (MONW). These folks have normal BMIs but display unhealthy characteristics typically associated with overweight, including reduced insulin sensitivity, greater total and visceral fat, and an inactive lifestyle.

In one small study, researchers in the department of nutrition at the University of Montreal wanted to find out which factors distinguish these "thin outside, fat inside" women from women with normal metabolisms. So they compared 12 women classified as MONW with 84 non-MONW women. They found that, compared with the non-MONW women, the small MONW group had higher body-fat percentages, higher levels of blood cholesterol, and less muscle. They were also less physically active and less likely to restrain their eating.

The Diabetes Lowdown

In 1994, doctors at East Carolina University School of Medicine in Greenville, North Carolina, who'd followed the progress of 608 severely obese people who had undergone weight-loss surgery at their hospital since 1980, noticed something startling.

The patients lost weight after the surgery, and 14 years later, 49 percent had kept it off. Amazingly, the 146 patients with type 2 diabetes and the 121 with impaired glucose tolerance, who had seen their blood sugar numbers improve days after surgery, *remained* virtually diabetes free.

Twenty years and dozens of studies later, in many cases, bariatric surgery resolved or significantly improved type 2 diabetes. In a 2004 analysis of 136 bariatric surgery studies that included 22,094 men and women—researchers found that type 2 diabetes disappeared completely in 76.8 percent of the patients who'd had the surgery.

"Patients with diabetes often see rapid improvements in their blood sugar levels after weight loss surgery, especially those who have gastric bypass," says Sherman Yu, MD, assistant professor of surgery at the University of Texas Medical School at Houston.

"We don't entirely understand why this happens, but the surgery appears to facilitate hormonal changes that help resolve diabetes."

All types of bariatric surgery involve reducing the size of the stomach so that it holds much less food. Typically, only people 100 or more pounds overweight, with serious obesity-related health problems are cleared for bariatric surgery. The surgery's risks include infection, blood clots, bowel obstructions, gallstones, and malnutrition. (The smaller digestive system cannot digest as many nutrients.)

Bottom line: If you're considering bariatric surgery, weigh the risks and benefits—and keep your expectations reasonable, says Ann L. Albright, PhD, RD, director of the Division of Diabetes Translation of the Centers for Disease Control and Prevention in Atlanta. "Bariatric surgery is a treatment for obesity, which can have very beneficial effects on type 2 diabetes," she says. "Unfortunately, a lot of people seeing patients for gastric bypass surgery are starting to use terms like 'reverse' and 'cure.' You have to be cautious about using terms like that, since an intensive nutrition plan must be followed after surgery."

There's no way to know for certain whether a relatively lean exterior conceals a fatty interior without undergoing a magnetic resonance imaging (MRI) or computed tomography (CT) scan, which allows scientists to see and quantify body fat. However, your answers to the questions below can help gauge your risk.

- Are you sedentary? Inactivity can lead to significant increases in visceral fat.

- Do you eat out of boxes, cans, and bags? Processed foods such as bakery goods, salty snacks, and fast foods tend to contain trans fats, an unhealthy fat linked to heart disease and, in test animals, excess abdominal fat.

- Do you smoke? Smokers have lower BMIs than nonsmokers, but they also have more abdominal fat. A study of more than 20,000 British men and women found that, compared with those who had never smoked, current smokers had bigger waist measurements.

Diabetes Rx

Perhaps you still think the odds of slimming down are stacked against you. Consider this encouraging news: Just trying to shed extra poundage may lengthen your life.

Researchers at the Centers for Disease Control and Prevention (CDC) followed 1,401 overweight diabetic people for 9 years. Those in the study who reported trying to lose weight had a 23 percent lower death rate than those who didn't, and the benefit was just as great for those who failed to shed pounds as for those who succeeded. One possible explanation: The "tryers" had adopted positive lifestyle habits, such as eating healthier foods and being more physically active. Though they didn't lose weight, they gained better health.

The point: Keep trying to shed those extra pounds—or those unhealthy habits. Especially if you have diabetes, the recommendations below can help.

■ **AIM LOW.** Set a goal to lose just 5 percent of your current body weight. A study conducted by the Diabetes Prevention Program, a landmark study of more than 3,000 men and women with prediabetes, found that those who reduced their body weight by just 7 percent—typically, 12 to 20 pounds—reduced their risk of diabetes by 58 percent over a 5-year period.

■ **GO WHOLE.** Swap processed and fast foods for foods in their natural state—such as fresh fruits and vegetables and whole grains—and you'll be on your way to a slimmer waistline and better health. Whole foods contain more fiber and healthy fats, which have been found to aid weight loss and help control blood sugar levels (see Take Advantage of Diabetes-Friendly Foods on page 339).

■ **TRIM TRANS FATS.** The American Heart Association recommends limiting consumption of trans fats to no more than 1 percent of daily calories. To meet that goal, you'll have to read beyond the label. Under current federal guidelines, a food with 0.4 grams of trans fats per serving can be listed as having zero trans fats. If the food is labeled "zero trans fat," check its ingredients list for "partially hydrogenated." If you see that term, the product contains some trans fats.

■ **GIVE YOURSELF A CUE.** Drape a tape measure over your towel rack, where you'll see it every day. This visual reminder will help stiffen your resolve to eat well and meet your 5 percent goal.

Measure your waistline once a week. For the most accurate measurement, place the tape around your bare abdomen just above your hip bone. Keep the tape snug—don't pull—and parallel to the floor. Relax, exhale, and measure.

■ **IF YOU SMOKE, QUIT.** People with type 2 diabetes who smoke risk nerve damage and kidney disease and are three times more likely to die of cardiovascular disease than nonsmokers with diabetes.

Quitting is tough, but you don't have to go it alone. Ask your doctor if

Weight-Loss Medication: The Straight Dope

We keep hoping for that magic weight-loss pill. Researchers studying the effects of weight-loss drugs keep delivering less-than-miraculous conclusions. The experts' consensus: Weight-loss medications can work, including for people with type 2 diabetes. However, they work best when they're teamed with a sensible eating plan and regular exercise.

In a 2005 study, University of Pennsylvania researchers divided 224 overweight men and women into four groups, gave them different combinations of weight-loss therapies—including the weight-loss drug sibutramine (Meridia)—and followed their progress for a year. Researchers told all the participants to consume 1,200 to 1,500 calories a day and exercise 30 minutes a day on most days.

Group 3, which teamed the medication with lifestyle modifications, lost the most weight: 26.6 pounds. Group 1 (sibutramine only) lost 11, group 2 (lifestyle modification only) lost 15, and group 4 (sibutramine and brief lifestyle counseling) lost 16.5 pounds.

In general, combining weight-loss medications with more physical activity and fewer calories can help you shed 5 to 10 percent of your body weight within a year. Besides sibutramine, currently available prescription medications include:

■ Phentermine (Adipex-P, Fastin, Ionamin, Obenix, Oby-trim, Phentercot, Phentride, Pro-Fast, Teramine, Zantryl)

quit-smoking medications such as bupropion (Zyban) or varenicline (Chantix) might be right for you. Or join a support group. Your company or health plan may sponsor a quit group. If not, call the nearest hospital or your local chapter of the American Lung Association or the American Cancer Society to see if they offer free or low-cost classes.

- Diethylpropion (Tenuate, Tepanil)

- Mazindol (Sanorex, Mazanor)

- Phendimetrazine (Adipost, Bontril, Melfiat, Obezine, Phendiet, Plegine, Prelu-2)

- Benzphetamine (Didrex)

- Orlistat (Xenical)

Most of these medications have been approved for short-term use—a few weeks or months. Sibutramine and Orlistat are the only weight-loss medications approved for longer-term use in obese patients, although their safety and effectiveness have not been established for use beyond 2 years.

Only your doctor can tell you which, if any, weight-loss medications are right for you, says Ann Albright, PhD, RD, director of the Division of Diabetes Translation for the Centers for Disease Control and Prevention in Atlanta. For example, if you have heart disease, high blood pressure, or liver or kidney disease, you may not be a good candidate, says Dr. Albright.

If you are prescribed these medications, you'll still need to monitor carbohydrate intake and portion sizes. "Just because you're on a weight-loss medication doesn't mean you can eat whatever you want, as some weight-loss medications advertised on TV say," says Dr. Albright. "That claim is untrue—and unconscionable. You still need to monitor caloric content and portion sizes."

■ **MAKE EXERCISE SHORT AND SWEET.** Commit to at least 30 minutes of physical activity 5 days a week. "Visceral fat is very sensitive to exercise," says Dr. Hamdy. Choose an activity you enjoy. Walk outdoors, dance, do yoga, or swim. The more fun you have, the more you're likely to stick with it.

6. Get the Healthiest Mix of Carbs, Protein, Fat, and Fiber

EACH DAY AT MERCY MEDICAL CENTER in Baltimore, Linda Yerardi, RD, CDE, helps those newly diagnosed with type 2 diabetes formulate their eating plans. But she's more than a certified diabetes educator. She's a myth-buster.

"My clients think I'm going to be the food police—'Sorry, you can't have this or this or this,'" says Yerardi. She loves to prove them wrong.

Recently, says Yerardi, one of her patients—a 6-foot-2 state trooper—sat in her office and said sadly, "I love Outback. Are you going to tell me that I can't eat there anymore? I need my Outback." Yerardi logged on to the national chain's Web site, which lists the nutrition information for each of its items, as well as diabetic and heart-healthy choices. "I said, 'Look. You can have the steak, the baked sweet potato, and the steamed veggies.' He was a happy man."

That tasty meal boasts more than flavor. It contains the perfect mix of the three main nutrients in food—carbohydrates, protein, and fat, collectively known as macronutrients—and fiber, the indigestible carbohydrate in plant foods with proven health benefits. All of these nutrients play a role in blood sugar control.

Trimmed of excess fat, the steak provides protein. With a pat of margarine or a drizzle of olive oil, the sweet potato supplies good-for-you complex carbohydrates, fats, and fiber. The steamed vegetables offer more good carbohydrates and fiber. Practice portion control and limit added fats such as butter, and it's a meal even a nutritionist can love.

There's no downside to planning your meals around the correct amounts of macronutrients and fiber. This strategy, which we call eating in balance, is good for both your blood sugar and your heart and can even help you lose weight. "Following a diet that's low in fat, moderate in carbohydrates and proteins, and high in fiber is a good goal for everyone, regardless of whether they have diabetes," says Yerardi.

In this chapter, you'll discover more about how these nutrients affect your blood sugar, why it's important to get the proper amounts of each, and how to select the healthiest sources. You'll also discover a simple way to eat in balance—every time.

The Benefits of Balance

There's a simple reason to plan your meals around proper amounts of macronutrients and fiber: pure satisfaction.

"When you eat in balance, you feel fuller and more satisfied," says Ann Fittante, RD, a registered dietitian and certified diabetes educator at the Joslin Diabetes Center education affiliate at Swedish Medical Center in Seattle. You're less likely to gorge at your next meal, she says, or to crave the sweets and starches that can wreak havoc on blood sugar and weight. And each macronutrient contributes to that I'm-full sensation.

Carbohydrates—either the complex carbohydrates in whole grains, fruits, and vegetables or the refined kind in white bread, white pasta, and white rice—all break down into blood glucose. However, they break down at different rates.

Because your body has to work hard to digest complex carbohydrates, they enter the bloodstream gradually, causing a slow, gentle rise in blood sugar. As a bonus, complex carbohydrates are also rich in *fiber,* and evidence suggests that a high-fiber diet promotes long-term glucose control in people with diabetes.

By contrast, your body digests refined carbohydrates quickly. As a result, their energy floods the bloodstream, causing blood sugar levels to soar. Phase refined carbohydrates out of your diet and replace them with complex carbohydrates and you'll eat healthier, have more energy, and find it easier to lose extra pounds.

Foods high in *protein,* such as eggs and egg whites, tofu, meat, poultry, fish, and dried or canned beans, have little effect on blood sugar because protein tends to slow the rate at which your body absorbs carbohydrate. Protein also has a high satiety factor—eating it satisfies your hunger longer.

Foods rich in *fat*—either from plant foods such as vegetable oils, nuts, and nut butters or animal foods such as meat, milk, and cheese—also don't significantly affect blood sugar. Fats, too, slow digestion and in turn delay the rise in blood sugar. At times, however, a very high-fat meal can slow the absorption process too much and keep blood-sugar levels higher than they should be for a longer period of time.

Just as you should consume the right amounts of these nutrients, you should also choose the right kinds. For example, the fiber-full complex carbohydrates in a bowl of oatmeal and berries will stick with you longer—and have a more positive effect on blood cholesterol and blood sugar—than the unhealthy carbs and fats in a jelly doughnut. Fiber-rich foods also tend to squash the cravings triggered by a steady diet of refined carbohydrates.

Now that you understand how these nutrients affect your blood glucose, you're ready to receive your "prescriptions" for each.

Carbohydrates: Pick the Premium Fuel

- Make carbohydrates 40 to 60 percent of your daily calories.

- Women: Get 30 to 60 grams of carbohydrate per meal, 15 grams per snack.

- Men: Get 30 to 75 grams of carbohydrate per meal, 15 grams per snack.

- Eat a minimum of 130 grams of carbohydrate per day.

The Diabetes Food Pyramid

More fruit, vegetables, and whole grains. Less fats, sweets, and alcohol. On those golden rules of nutrition, the USDA food pyramid for the general public (MyPyramid) and the pyramid designed for people with type 2 diabetes (the Diabetes Food Pyramid) agree.

However, the Diabetes Food Pyramid is based on carbohydrates' significant effects on blood sugar. Here's what you need to know.

The Diabetes Food Pyramid groups foods based on their carbohydrate and protein content, not on their classification as a food. Both pyramids split foods into six categories. But the Diabetes Food Pyramid places cheese in its meat-and-other-proteins group and beans in its breads-grains-and-other-starches group. MyPyramid has cheese in its milk group and groups beans with meat.

The Diabetes Food Pyramid bases a food's serving size on its carbohydrate content. In the diabetes pyramid, ⅓ cup of pasta or rice or ¾ cup of ready-to-eat cereal is 1 serving. In MyPyramid, ½ cup of pasta or rice or 1 cup of dry cereal constitutes 1 serving.

Both pyramids recommend a range of serving sizes for each group. In general, most women need the lowest number of servings in each food group (about 1,600 calories a day). Very active men may need the maximum number of servings (about 2,800 calories a day). "Choose your number of servings carefully, especially if you need to lose weight," says Linda Yerardi, RD, CDE, a certified diabetes educator at Mercy Medical Center in Baltimore.

The Diabetes Food Pyramid gives you a solid overview of a healthy diet if you have diabetes, says Yerardi—but don't stop there. "If you have diabetes, work with a health provider to create a meal plan based on your unique needs, and that includes your favorite foods," she says. To learn more about the Diabetes Food Pyramid, log on to the American Diabetes Association Web site at diabetes.org.

Cars run on gas. Humans run on carbohydrate—it's our preferred source of fuel. Nutrient-rich and fiber-packed, complex carbohydrates burn "cleaner" than refined carbohydrates. As a result, we run better—have more energy, fewer cravings, and better blood sugar control. We tend to stay slimmer, too.

Each human body is a unique machine, and each requires varying amounts of carbohydrates to run at its peak. The optimal amount depends on weight, age, activity level, and other factors. In general, however, carbohydrates should make up from 40 to 60 percent of your daily calories. That means if you consume 1,500 calories a day, 600 to 900 of them should come from carbohydrates.

Fittante prefers to think in terms of carbohydrates per meal rather than a daily percentage. Women with type 2 diabetes can typically consume from 30 to 60 grams of carbohydrate per meal and 15 per snack, she says. Most men with diabetes can handle 30 to 75 grams of carbohydrate per meal and 15 per snack. To keep your energy high, don't drop below 130 grams of carbohydrate a day.

Grains and grain products are our primary source of carbohydrates, so it's important to select the most nutrition-packed varieties. Because whole grains pack more vitamins, minerals, fiber, and health-promoting plant chemicals than processed grains, experts recommend making half of your daily grain servings whole grains or foods made from them.

While making the switch from refined to complex carbs may take some getting used to, the benefits to blood sugar, heart health, and weight control are enormous. Some swaps are simple: Trade white rice for brown. Replace pasta, breads, and cereals made with white flour with whole grain varieties. (You can start with half whole grain pasta and half white pasta.) Explore your local natural-foods store for more exotic whole grains, such as bulgur, wheat berries, amaranth, and quinoa and whole grain breads, crackers, tortillas, and breakfast cereals. Add dried beans and lentils to your soups, chili, and stews—they're an excellent source of fiber.

However, even healthy carbohydrates can push up blood sugar levels and add extra calories when they're eaten in too-large quantities, so watch how much you dish out. Later on in this chapter, you'll learn a portion-control method that works every time.

Fiber: Part of the Healthy-Carb Package

- Consume 14 grams of fiber for every 1,000 calories you eat each day, or a minimum of 20 grams each day.

Your mother called it roughage. Scientists call it dietary fiber—the parts of plant foods that pass through our bodies undigested. Hundreds of studies link a high-fiber diet with a reduced risk of heart disease and, it's been suggested, improved glucose control. The best part: When you switch over to healthy carbs, the fiber's thrown in for free.

Dietary fiber generally is characterized as insoluble or soluble in water. *Insoluble fiber,* the kind that provides "bulk," doesn't dissolve in water but aids digestion by speeding food through the stomach and intestines. Brown rice, most vegetables, whole grain cereals, and the skins of fruits are good sources of insoluble fiber.

Found in oatmeal, beans, and apples, *soluble fiber* soaks up water like a sponge, turns to a sticky goo in the intestines, and slows digestion, which delays the rise of blood sugar. Soluble fiber has been proven to lower total and "bad" LDL cholesterol and to improve blood sugar levels over the long term.

Experts recommend that adults consume 14 grams of fiber for every 1,000 calories they consume each day. That means if you typically stick to a 1,500-calorie-a-day diet, you should aim for 21 grams of fiber a day. You need both soluble and insoluble for optimum health. To get enough of each, eat a wide variety of plant foods.

Add fiber to your diet gradually, over a few weeks' time. That way, you'll avoid digestive distress such as abdominal bloating, cramping, and gas. Drink plenty of water, too—up to ten 8-ounce glasses daily—to help move all that fiber through your system.

Proteins: Less (and Lean) Is More

■ Keep protein intake to 15 to 20 percent of total calories.

If you're a committed carnivore, you're not alone. People with diabetes don't need to give up red meat any more than they need to avoid chocolate. For the sake of your heart, however, it's wise to broaden your definition of protein.

Perhaps because the United States is the richest country in the world, we've always made red meat our primary source of protein. Yet meat, along with our other primary proteins—poultry, seafood, eggs, and cheese—is not comprised solely of protein. These foods also contain fats, both saturated and unsaturated, in varying amounts.

Dried beans, lentils, and some grains contain good amounts of protein and virtually no fat of any kind but are often categorized as carbohydrates because that is their predominant nutrient. Other recommended sources of lean protein include fish, skinless poultry, tofu, and fat-free or low-fat dairy products. Higher-fat cuts of beef, pork, or lamb, as well as high-fat dairy products, should be eaten only occasionally.

If you love meat, there's no need to give it up. Simply eat smaller servings—1 to 2 ounces per meal—several times a week instead of every day. To stretch your meat budget, incorporate small amounts into a main dish rather than making meat the focus of your meal. For example, flavor tomato sauce with a small amount of low-fat ground beef. Fill homemade burritos with brown rice and beans instead of beef. Add a few ounces of stir-fried lean beef, fish, or chicken breast to tender-crisp veggies and serve it over wild rice. These tips conform to the eating-in-balance principles—more complex carbs and fiber, less fat.

Fats: Easy (and Healthy) Does It

■ Keep intake of total fat to 30 to 35 percent predominantly healthy fats.

■ Limit saturated fats to less than 7 percent of total calories.

- Eat two servings of fish per week.

- Limit daily intake of dietary cholesterol to 200 milligrams or less.

In the 1980s, a kind of nutritional Dark Ages, the nation gorged on low-fat everything—and gained weight. Your body needs the right kinds of fat in the right amounts to stay healthy and function at its peak.

Dietary fats generally are characterized as saturated and unsaturated. Unhealthy *saturated fats* raise blood cholesterol, clog blood vessels, stiffen cell membranes, and drive up blood pressure. Sources of saturated fats include high-fat red meat such as regular ground beef, sausage, and spareribs and whole-fat dairy products such as milk, cheese, and ice cream. Foods high in saturated fats, along with egg yolks, are typically high in dietary *cholesterol*.

Structurally similar to saturated fats, *trans fats* lurk in processed and fast foods and stick margarine. Some researchers suspect that trans fats raise total cholesterol even more than saturated fats do. They also tend to raise LDL cholesterol and lower levels of "good" HDL cholesterol and have similar unhealthy effects on blood glucose.

To help protect your heart, replace these unhealthy fats with *unsaturated fats*. The two types of unsaturated fats, monounsaturated and polyunsaturated, don't raise total or LDL cholesterol and may even help lower LDL cholesterol. Olive oil, nuts, and nut butters are rich in monounsaturated fats, shown to reduce triglyceride levels, and may also improve control of blood glucose. Walnuts, pumpkin or sunflower seeds, and safflower, soybean, and sunflower oils are good sources of polyunsaturated fats.

Put fish on your plate, too. Salmon, albacore tuna, and other cold-water fish are rich in heart-protective *omega-3 fatty acids*. In one study, women with diabetes who regularly ate fish or other foods high in omega-3s, such as walnuts or flaxseed oil, had lower rates of heart disease.

If you haven't tried the margarines that help lower total and LDL cholesterol (such as Promise Activ and Benecol), give them a shot. Their plant

The Diabetes Lowdown

If you have type 2 diabetes, perhaps you use the glycemic index—a system that ranks the effects of carbohydrates such as bread, fruits, veggies, and sweets on blood sugar—to guide your food choices. But a recent University of South Carolina study suggested that eating "low GI" may not cut your blood sugar. So is the glycemic index still a valid tool with which to manage your blood sugar?

Yes, says Ann Fittante, RD, a registered dietitian and certified diabetes educator at the Joslin Diabetes Center education affiliate at Swedish Medical Center in Seattle. "You can't write off the GI because of one study," she says.

The study, which relied on food questionnaires from 1,255 men and women, assessed their intake of high-glycemic foods (such as watermelon and white bread) and low-glycemic foods (such as bran cereal and low-fat yogurt). Researchers tested the volunteers' blood sugar levels twice during the 5-year study and found no significant correlation between the glycemic index of foods and the subjects' blood-sugar levels.

Many factors can affect the impact of food on blood sugar, including the length of time that food is cooked and other foods eaten at the same time. Also, some low-GI foods, such as peanut M&M's, pack more sugar, fat, and calories than some high-GI foods, such as steamed carrots.

That's why you don't want to use the GI system as your only meal-planning tool. If you do, you might overdo the low-fat ice cream and M&M's, which sit low on the glycemic index, and eat less watermelon and whole grain cereal, which are high-GI foods.

GI experts have always said that controlling calories and portion size and choosing more fruits, vegetables, and whole grains over refined carbs is the essence of low-GI eating, but it's not clear whether the people in the study took all of these steps. What's more, hundreds of studies show that eating in this healthy, moderate way is an effective way to control blood sugar, lose weight, and keep the pounds off.

"If you use the GI as a meal-planning tool now, and your blood sugar is in target, it's fine to continue to use it," says Fittante. Bottom line: If it ain't broke, don't fix it.

stanols or sterols block the absorption of the cholesterol in food, making them a healthy alternative to the unhealthy fats in butter and stick margarine. They're available in the dairy section of most supermarkets.

Remember, even healthy fats such as olive oil and nuts are high in calories, so keep tabs on how much you use if you're trying to lose weight.

Create the Perfect Plate—Every Meal

Maybe you know a child who eats from one of those sectioned dishes so the corn won't touch the mashed potatoes. (Maybe you even used one yourself.) You can borrow the idea to ensure that you eat the optimum amounts of healthy carbs, good fats, lean protein, and fiber at each meal. The "plate method" helps you stay on track with your nutrient prescription—and it'll help you eat sensible portions, too, says Fittante. Here's how to use it.

■ **START WITH A 9-INCH DINNER PLATE.** Plates with the diameter of a hubcap—like those used in most restaurants—will inflate your portion sizes. If you own supersized platters, scale down to petite plates.

■ **PRACTICE SIMPLE DIVISION.** Each time you sit down to a meal, imagine a vertical line that divides the center of your plate. Then draw an imaginary line to divide one half of your plate into two quarters.

■ **PORTION OUT THE CARBS.** Fill one-fourth of your plate with grains (more often than not, whole grains) or starchy veggies such as potatoes, corn, or peas. "That translates to a cup of rice, pasta, or cereal; a medium potato; or two pieces of whole grain bread," says Fittante.

■ **ADD PROTEIN.** Fill the other quarter of your plate with protein, either from an animal source or a vegetable source such as tofu or beans. If you're eating meat, trim away all visible fat. Remove skin from chicken or turkey. Hold the fatty sauces and gravies, too.

■ **FINISH WITH FIBER.** Fill the remaining half of your plate with nonstarchy vegetables—salad brimming with tomatoes, red and yellow peppers, red onions, and cucumbers or roasted, grilled, or steamed veggies such as carrots, broccoli, or cauliflower.

■ **TRACK ADDED FAT.** A drizzle of olive oil for your salad, a pat of heart-healthy spread made with vegetable oil, or a small amount of low-fat mayo or low-fat sour cream is okay.

■ **REFILL THE RIGHT WAY.** Ideally, you'll fill your plate once at each meal, says Yerardi. After a meal, if you're still hungry, refill the half of your plate reserved for salad or cooked vegetables, she says. If you're still hungry after that, refill the quarter of your plate reserved for protein.

One more thing. If you use insulin, "you still need to count carbohydrates or exchanges in meals to make sure your medications are keeping your blood glucose on target," says Ann Albright, PhD, RD, director of the Division of Diabetes Translation for the Centers for Disease Control and Prevention in Atlanta.

7. Take Advantage of Diabetes-Friendly Foods

IN THE PAST FEW YEARS, doctors and researchers have made huge strides in the treatment of type 2 diabetes. Yet one simple, natural method stands out from the rest: food. Armed with the simple dietary guidelines in the last chapter, you can customize a menu that trims your waistline, balances your blood sugar, and pleases your palate.

As you tweak your eating plan, make sure to include the foods below. Research suggests that these foods help prevent type 2 diabetes and its complications.

A Whole Lot of Healthy: Whole Grains

In a 2006 survey of 1,040 adults, 41 percent said they were eating more whole grains than they did the year before. That's great news. Packed with nutrients and wrapped in a high-fiber coating, whole grains are a perfect nutritional package.

If you're concerned about managing your blood sugar or diabetes-related complications, it's time to heed the whole grain message. A diet rich in whole grains reduces the risk of diabetes, research shows, but it gets even better.

Studies have revealed that just three servings of whole grains a day also can help improve blood sugar control in people already diagnosed with diabetes and keep arteries wide open and supple, thereby warding off heart attack and stroke.

Whole grains, the seeds of various grass plants, provide important nutrients and fiber. Each of the three parts of a seed plays a role in nourishing you.

- Bran: The outer layer of the skin of the wheat seed is a rich source of vitamins and minerals, including B vitamins and fiber.

- Germ: Designed to nourish the new wheat plant after it sprouts, the germ contains healthy fats, plant chemicals, and minerals such as magnesium, which helps the body break down carbohydrates and control insulin. In two large Harvard studies, people who consumed the most magnesium in their diets significantly lowered their risk of type 2 diabetes.

- Endosperm: The starchy core of grains contains mostly protein and carbohydrates and smaller amounts of B vitamins.

Refined grains, used to make white bread and pasta, have had their nutrient-rich bran and germ stripped away. In fact, all-purpose flour is mostly the endosperm.

Whole grains' cornucopia of nutrients includes more than fiber, however. "The individual components of whole grains have an additive and synergistic effect," says Joanne Slavin, PhD, professor in the department of food science and nutrition at the University of Minnesota and an expert on the health benefits of whole grains. "It's the combination and interactions between components that we believe provide the protection against disease."

Diabetes Rx

- **BE WHOLE-HEARTED.** Make at least half of your daily grain servings whole grains. It's easier than you think. Choose oatmeal or whole grain cereal for breakfast, whole wheat bread for your lunchtime sandwich, half a cup of brown rice for dinner, and a cup of air-popped popcorn with your evening sitcoms, and you're there.

■ **LEARN THE LABEL LINGO.** More often than not, those "multigrain" crackers or that "stone-ground" loaf contains mostly refined white flour. To your body, that's the same as sugar. To know if it's really a whole grain food, check each product's ingredients list and apply the rules below.

- Wheat and rye: If you don't see the word *whole*, the product is made from refined wheat flour.

- Oats: Whether you see the word *whole* or not, you're getting whole oats.

- Corn: Look for the word *whole*.

■ **CUSTOMIZE YOUR CARBS.** Eating more whole grains may raise the amount of carbohydrate in your diet, which could affect your blood sugar. If you take medication for type 2 diabetes, your doctor may need to adjust it. You may also need to space your whole grain servings throughout the day to keep your blood sugar in balance.

Use Your Bean: Legumes

Beans may never live down their reputation as the musical fruit, but they sure are healthy—versatile, too. You can cook up a savory stew from the tiny but hearty lentil; top brown rice with smoky black beans; and turn garbanzos into the tangy Mediterranean spread hummus. No matter which variety you choose, beans benefit blood sugar, blood fats, and body weight.

Beans are high in soluble fiber, the same gummy stuff in oatmeal shown to lower levels of total blood cholesterol. One cooked cup can provide as much as 17 grams, more than half of the 24 grams recommended daily for women. Fiber fills you up, too, which can help control your appetite—and weight.

Beans also sit low on the glycemic index, which means they produce a slow, gradual rise in blood sugar, desirable for people with type 2 diabetes.

The heart loves beans, too. Virtually fat free, with zero cholesterol, they are also rich in the B vitamin folate. Research suggests that folate may help lower elevated blood levels of homocysteine, an amino acid that may damage the arteries and raise the risk of heart disease and stroke.

Beans are also a rich but overlooked source of potent antioxidants called flavonoids, found in berries and wine. The darker the bean, the more flavonoids it contains.

Diabetes Rx

■ **AIM FOR ⅓ CUP A DAY.** Researchers from Harvard University's School of Public Health compared 2,118 men and women in Costa Rica who'd had heart attacks with an equal number of heart-healthy people. Those who ate ⅓ cup of beans a day were 38 percent less likely to have suffered a heart attack than those who ate beans less than once a month.

■ **ADD BLACK BEANS TO YOUR MENU.** Popular in Latin American cuisine, the small, glossy black turtle bean often finds its way into burritos, soups, and chili. Researchers at the University of Guelph in Ontario tested the antioxidant powers of flavonoids in the skin of 12 common dry beans. Black beans contained the most flavonoids, followed by red, brown, yellow, and white beans. A particular kind of flavonoid called anthocyanin was the most active antioxidant in the black beans. The researchers noted that although their study tested dry beans, frozen or canned ones may pack a similar antioxidant punch.

Just Say Moo: Low-Fat Dairy

When you were a kid, your mother told you that milk was good for your growing bones. As it turns out, low-fat, calcium-rich dairy foods in general appear to be good for people at risk for type 2 diabetes. Studies suggest that increased dairy intake may have positive effects on insulin resistance, blood pressure, heart health, and body weight.

What's more, a multi-university study found that women who regularly consumed low-fat dairy foods lowered their risk of type 2 diabetes by more than 20 percent. Researchers led by Brigham and Women's Hospital in Boston analyzed data on more than 37,000 women (average age: mid-50s). At the study's start, none had diabetes. The women completed surveys about their eating habits, which covered more than 100 foods and beverages, including fat-free and whole milk, yogurt, cheese, and cottage cheese. The women were followed for a decade, on average. During that time, 1,603 of them were diagnosed with diabetes.

After adjusting for factors such as weight, fiber consumption, physical activity, and family history of diabetes, women with the highest intake of dairy foods were 21 percent less likely to develop type 2 than those with the lowest intake. In fact, each serving-per-day increase in dairy intake was associated with a 4-percent lower risk. Other studies have linked low-fat dairy consumption and lowered diabetes risk in men.

Researchers don't know exactly how dairy products lower type 2 diabetes risk. But milk sugar (lactose) is converted to blood sugar at a relatively slow rate, which is good for blood sugar control and reducing insulin levels. We know that protein helps fill you up. And the fat even in low-fat dairy may help satisfy hunger, too.

Diabetes Rx

■ **CHOOSE LOW-FAT OR FAT-FREE FARE.** Low-fat or fat-free yogurt, milk, cottage cheese, and cheeses are better for heart health. If you haven't tried low-fat cheeses in a while, give them another try. They've come a long way—the quality and taste are better than ever.

■ **DO DAIRY WITHOUT DISTRESS.** If you're lactose intolerant, you can still get your diabetes-proofing dairy. Drink lactose-free milk, or opt for yogurt. (Enzymes in yogurt digest milk sugar for you.) Soy milk is another option. Most supermarkets carry several different brands and flavors.

Creamy, Crunchy Diabetes Busters: Nuts and Nut Butters

You perceive sneaking a few spoonfuls of peanut butter from the jar or a handful of nuts from the can as a guilty pleasure. Researchers view it as a heart-healthy habit.

Nuts have long been associated with reduced risk of heart disease, largely due to their ability to lower total and LDL cholesterol without lowering the "good" HDL variety. They are also proven to protect against type 2 diabetes. Harvard researchers who studied 84,000 women for 16 years found that those who ate $\frac{1}{4}$ cup of any nuts or 1 tablespoon of peanut butter at least five times a week reduced their risk of type 2 diabetes by 27 and 21 percent, respectively.

There are several ways nuts might put the crunch on type 2. Their rich amounts of monounsaturated fats may build healthier "skin" around cells, creating more efficient doorways for blood sugar to enter. Nuts' fiber and magnesium appear to help manage insulin levels, and their vitamins, minerals, antioxidants, and plant proteins may pitch in for healthy blood sugar and insulin regulation.

Feel free to swap peanuts or peanut butter for walnuts, pistachios, or almonds or almond or cashew butters. Peanuts and some nuts share a similar nutrition makeup, so the diabetes-fighting benefits should be similar for all of them.

Diabetes Rx

■ **PRACTICE PORTION PATROL.** Yes, nuts and nut butters are high in calories. (One tablespoon of peanut butter contains 95 calories; 1 ounce of nuts, 165 calories.) But you won't gain weight if you watch your serving and portion sizes. Researchers at Pennsylvania State University who studied peanut consumption in more than 14,000 people found that although nut and peanut butter eaters consumed more calories than those who ate fewer servings, their body mass index (BMI) scores were lower.

■ **MAKE SMART SWAPS.** To indulge without unwanted pounds, trade one serving of nuts or nut butter for equal amounts of calories from less-than-healthy foods, such as cookies or packaged snacks.

Smooth(ie) Out Blood Sugar: Soy Yogurt

Made by fermenting soy milk with the health-promoting bacteria added to many dairy yogurts, soy yogurt is a sweet and creamy treat that boasts the cholesterol-lowering benefits of soybeans. Now there's some evidence that soy yogurt—especially with blueberries or other fruit—contains active natural compounds that could play a role in managing type 2 diabetes.

Researchers at the University of Massachusetts at Amherst went to a local market and bought peach, strawberry, blueberry, and plain dairy yogurt made by four different manufacturers. They also bought one brand of soy yogurt in the same four flavors. Then they analyzed extracts from all the yogurts for specific properties that could help control type 2 diabetes and high blood pressure.

Specifically, they tested the yogurts' ability to inhibit three enzymes. The first two: alpha-amylase and alpha-glucosidase, which help break down carbohydrates into blood sugar. Blocking their effects slows the digestion of carbohydrates, thereby lengthening the time it takes for blood sugar to rise after a meal. (Diabetes medications called alpha-glucosidase inhibitors target these same enzymes.) The researchers also tested the yogurts' ability to inhibit angiotensin-I converting enzyme (ACE-1), which causes blood vessels to narrow, raising blood pressure.

The yogurts were also tested for their antioxidant activity—phenolic compounds, in particular, which in some studies blocked the action of alpha-amylase. These plant chemicals give dark-hued vegetables and fruits—including berries—their health benefits.

Soy yogurt with blueberries was the clear winner: It inhibited all three enzymes tested. Peach and strawberry soy yogurts inhibited two: alpha-amylase and alpha-glucosidase.

Soy yogurt—even the nonfruited variety—contained the highest amounts of phenolic compounds and the most antioxidant activity, with blueberry dairy yogurts as the runners-up. Both blueberry yogurts also blocked the action of alpha-glucosidase the best.

As for blocking ACE-1, soy yogurts did the best job, and they also had the highest phenolic phytochemical content overall.

Diabetes Rx

■ **EXERCISE FREE CHOICE.** The researchers used Whole Soy brand yogurt in their study, but you can find Silk Live!, Stonyfield Farms, and other soy yogurts at supermarkets and natural-foods stores.

■ **GO FOR THE BLUE.** Since blueberries pack the most phenolic compounds, it makes sense to opt for blueberry soy yogurt. But the other varieties may still provide some blood sugar benefits.

■ **CONSIDER YOUR CARBS.** Though healthy, soy yogurt is fairly high in carbohydrates, so you'll need to consider its effect on your blood sugar if you have type 2 diabetes. A 6-ounce serving of a fruited soy yogurt contains 27 to 32 grams of carbohydrate, about the amount in two slices of bread or a medium banana. The nutrition content of many fruited dairy yogurts is similar.

A Mug o' Protection: Coffee

Several studies have associated heavy coffee intake (5 or more cups a day) with improved sensitivity to insulin and a lower risk for type 2 diabetes. But what if you drink just 2 cups or prefer decaf or instant? Can you still reap the benefits of the bean?

It appears so. Researchers at the Harvard School of Public Health wanted to know if smaller amounts of coffee would reduce type 2 diabetes risk and if decaffeinated and instant coffee would have the same protective effect as the full-strength, slow-drip brew. So they examined 88,259 women's intake of coffee and other caffeine-containing foods and drinks in 3 separate years. Their analysis included different types and amounts of coffee.

The Diabetes Lowdown

Charlotte Hayes, a certified diabetes educator in Atlanta, recalls a TV ad for a brand of bars and shakes created for people with type 2 diabetes. As a middle-aged couple strolls on a beach, we're told that these products help them manage their blood sugar and protect their health.

Although the couple was barefoot—not a great idea for folks with diabetes—these products have a place in diabetes management. "People are eating more and more on the run, and these products are convenient," says Hayes. "They're calorie- and portion-controlled and need no refrigeration." Their slow-digesting carbohydrates, including fiber and resistant starch, help minimize peaks in blood sugar.

What these bars and shakes are not: food. "Whole, real food is always the better choice," says Hayes. "There are so many health-promoting substances in fruits, vegetables, and whole grains—some we haven't even discovered yet. Manufactured foods don't have those."

Her advice: Save the bars and shakes for when it's inconvenient or impossible to eat a healthy meal: at the airport, on a long flight, or during a hectic day. Or make your own meal replacements. "Combine a handful of whole grain cereal with some nuts and dried fruit, and you've got trail mix," she says. (Watch your portions—a handful or two is enough.) Other grab-and-go options: fruit or an almond-butter or turkey sandwich on whole grain bread.

When using diabetic bars and beverages, follow these guidelines.

- Test your blood sugar after consuming a diabetes bar or drink for the first time. Each product has a unique formulation, and its glycemic effect may also be unique.

- Use these products only as occasional meal replacements, or fit them into a meal as a carbohydrate choice.

- If you use insulin or insulin secretagogues (medications that stimulate the pancreas to secrete more insulin), don't use these products to treat low blood sugar. They may not raise blood glucose quickly enough. Instead, carry mini boxes of raisins or some hard candy, which will raise blood sugar fast.

After 10 years, 1,263 of the women had developed diabetes. The researchers found that drinking 1 cup of coffee a day reduced the risk of type 2 diabetes by 13 percent; 2 to 3 cups, 42 percent; and 4 or more, 47 percent.

But consider this: Coffee's positive effects were not due to its caffeine. The study's lead author, Rob M. van Dam, PhD, suspects that a component in coffee beans called chlorogenic acid might play a role. Studies of human cells suggest that chlorogenic acid can inhibit the secretion of glucose in the liver. If the substance does that in a coffee drinker, "it could reduce glucose levels in the blood and offer a quite plausible hypothesis for coffee's apparent protective effect" against type 2 diabetes, says Dr. van Dam.

Diabetes Rx

■ **AVOID MEGACALORIE COFFEEHOUSE OFFERINGS.** Those exotic flavored syrups and towers of whipped cream can add hundreds of calories to your cuppa. Drink too many, and you could gain weight, undoing coffee's protective effects. Opt for regular coffee with fat-free milk (your best choice) or a dribble of half-and-half, and hold the sugar.

CONSIDER DECAF. If you have type 2 diabetes, high blood pressure, or heart disease, choose decaf, which will reduce potentially negative effects on blood pressure.

Tonic in a Teacup: Green Tea

Perhaps you prefer the delicate flavor of green tea to coffee—you're in luck. Your favorite brew may also help protect against type 2 diabetes.

Researchers in Japan wanted to know whether there is a connection between consumption of green tea and the risk for type 2 diabetes and—if so—whether caffeine fully accounts for this link. They used questionnaires from 17,413 men and women—already gathered as a part of a large national cancer study in Japan—that included information about their health, lifestyle, and consumption of tea and coffee. At that time, none of the participants said they had type 2 diabetes. Five years later, when they repeated the questionnaire, 444 men and women reported that they'd developed type 2.

Compared with those who drank less than a cup of green tea a week, those who drank 6 cups or more a day—or 3 or more cups of coffee—were about one-third less likely to develop type 2 diabetes. Green tea's effect was stronger in women than in men.

Green tea is rich in catechins, plant substances with potent antioxidant compounds. Test-tube studies have shown that the catechin epigallocatechin gallate (EGCG) accounts for most of green tea's beneficial effects on insulin.

Diabetes Rx

■ **SIP A CUP SEVERAL TIMES A DAY.** Much of the research documenting the health benefits of green tea is based on the amount of green tea typically consumed in Asian countries—about 3 cups per day. Sipping throughout the day will help your body absorb its healthful plant substances without interfering with the absorption of iron in fruits and vegetables.

■ **STEEP WELL.** Allow the tea to steep for 5 minutes to get the full benefits of its catechins.

Vinegar: A Spoonful Helps the Sugar Go Down

Start your next meal with a salad bursting with fresh veggies. Dress it with vinegar, and you may benefit your blood sugar even more.

Arizona State University researchers broke 29 test subjects into three groups. The first group had type 2 diabetes; the second, prediabetes. The third group was healthy. The researchers fed everyone a high-carbohydrate breakfast of orange juice and a bagel with butter. Before the meal, the subjects were given either 2 tablespoons of apple cider vinegar or a placebo. A week later, the groups switched—the vinegar group received the placebo and vice versa—but ate the same breakfast.

The vinegar improved postmeal blood sugar levels in all three groups. But those with prediabetes benefited most: Their blood sugar levels dropped 34

THE DIABETES FOOD FOE

As you add diabetes-friendly foods to your menu, limit fast foods, packaged snacks, and baked goodies. These processed foods contain trans fats, which research suggests may promote heart disease and even health-threatening belly fat.

Formed when vegetable oils used to manufacture foods undergo a process called hydrogenation, trans fats raise levels of "bad" LDL cholesterol, lower levels of "good" HDL cholesterol, and increase the tendency of blood platelets to clump and form artery-clogging clots. Trans fats may also cause inflammation, a "hyperactivity" of the immune system. Left unchecked, low-grade inflammation might be a factor in the development of diabetes, heart disease, and other serious health conditions.

A Harvard University study of almost 33,000 women found that those with the highest intake of these fats—about 3.6 grams a day—had triple the risk of heart disease, compared with women who consumed the least (2.5 grams). It's estimated that the average daily American diet contains about 5.8 grams of trans fat.

In animal studies, trans fats have been linked to belly fat. Researchers at Wake Forest University School of Medicine in Winston-Salem, North Carolina, divided 42 monkeys into two groups. The first group got 8 percent of their calories from trans fat—comparable, researchers said, to the amount consumed by people who eat a lot of fried food. The second group got 8 percent of their calories as monounsaturated fat, the kind found in heart-healthy olive oil and nuts. Both groups of monkeys consumed the same overall number of calories.

After 6 years on the diet, the trans fat–fed monkeys had gained 7.2 percent of their body weight, compared with 1.8 percent in the unsaturated group. The kicker: Computed tomography (CT) scans showed that the trans fat monkeys carried 30 percent more abdominal fat. "We were shocked," says lead researcher Kylie Kavanagh, DVM. "Despite our efforts to make sure they didn't gain weight, they still did. And most of that weight ended up on their tummies."

percent. Those with type 2 diabetes reduced their levels by about 20 percent with the vinegar. Vinegar contains a substance called acetic acid, "which may inhibit enzymes that digest starch," says lead researcher Carol Johnston, PhD. "So the carbohydrate molecules aren't available for absorption."

In fact, "vinegar appears to have effects similar to some of the most popular medications for diabetes," acarbose or metformin, says Dr. Johnston. "There are also studies suggesting that if people with prediabetes take these medications, they might reduce their chances of getting diabetes." If you take diabetes medication, consult your doctor before adding vinegar to your diet—and don't discontinue your medication.

Diabetes Rx

■ **STICK WITH THE RIGHT RATIO.** To reap vinegar's potential benefits, use at least 2 tablespoons of vinegar, as the study's participants did, says Dr. Johnston.

■ **OPT FOR THE REAL THING, NOT SUPPLEMENTS.** Although you can find commercially available vinegar dietary supplements, these products don't appear to contain acetic acid, says Dr. Johnston.

■ **ENJOY YOUR FAVORITE VINEGAR VARIETY.** Vinegars other than the apple cider variety contain 5 percent acetic acid, says Dr. Johnston, so feel free to enjoy your favorite: balsamic, red wine, or white.

8. Use Supplements Sensibly

LIKE MOST PRACTITIONERS of conventional medicine, Ryan Bradley, ND, "prescribes" a healthy diet and regular exercise for his patients with type 2 diabetes. If necessary, he adds medication.

Unlike most doctors, however, Dr. Bradley—a naturopathic physician who supervises the Diabetes and Cardiovascular Wellness Program at Bastyr University's Center for Natural Health in Seattle—rounds out his treatment plans with supplements. Combined with lifestyle changes, supplementation offers "consistent results on a regular basis," he says.

The herbs, vitamins, and minerals discussed below have been found to help manage diabetes and its complications in a variety of ways, research has found. Some of these supplements help lower blood sugar and improve insulin sensitivity. Others lower blood fats or help treat the complications of diabetes, including diabetic neuropathy.

Diabetes Rx

Before you take any supplement, follow these guidelines.

■ **CONSULT YOUR DOC.** When you have diabetes, it's best not to take any supplement until you discuss it with your doctor, says Dr. Bradley. Even natural substances can interact with prescription medications for diabetes. If you're taking medications to lower your blood sugar, some natural substances found to lower blood sugar may cause it to plummet dangerously.

■ **START SMALL.** To be on the safe side, start with half the recommended dosage and work up to a full dose over a week or so. Don't take more than the dosage instructions recommend.

■ **CONTINUE YOUR PRESCRIPTION MEDS.** Also, monitor your blood sugar while using the supplement, so you'll know if these supplements affect your numbers.

Acetyl-L-Carnitine

■ **WHAT IT IS:** Found naturally in the brain, liver, and kidneys, this molecule is structurally similar to the amino acid carnitine and plays a role in converting food into energy.

■ **WHAT WE KNOW:** Acetyl-L-carnitine has shown promise in the treatment of diabetic neuropathy, a condition that develops when high levels of sugar in the blood damage delicate nerve endings. The result is a stabbing, tingling, and burning pain in the legs, feet, and hands, especially at night.

Researchers at Wayne State University School of Medicine in Detroit evaluated the results of two studies testing two doses of acetyl-L-carnitine: 500 milligrams and 1,000 milligrams three times a day. Both studies, which involved a total of 1,257 people with diabetic neuropathy, lasted for 1 year. The researchers found that acetyl-L-carnitine reduced pain, improved sensory perception, and even appeared to help nerve fibers regenerate. Those who received 1,000 milligrams at a time tended to fare better than those who received the smaller amount.

■ **WHAT TO TAKE/DOSAGES:** Typical dosages for diabetic neuropathy range from 500 to 1,000 milligrams three times a day.

Alpha-Lipoic Acid

■ **WHAT IT IS:** Alpha-lipoic acid is an antioxidant made in the body. Working with other antioxidants, such as vitamins C and E, ALA attacks free radicals—waste products created when the body converts food into energy. Some experts believe that ALA is more powerful than vitamins E or C.

■ **WHAT WE KNOW:** Some studies have shown that ALA speeds the removal of sugar from a diabetic person's blood, possibly by lowering insulin levels and increasing the transport of sugar into cells. "ALA works especially well with exercise," says Dr. Bradley.

In Germany, ALA is a prescription drug used to treat diabetic neuropathy. A study between researchers at the Mayo Clinic and a medical center in Russia found that ALA significantly reduces the frequency and severity of symptoms of the most common kind of diabetic neuropathy. "It is known that ALA is a very strong antioxidant," says Peter J. Dyck, MD, professor of neurology at the Mayo Clinic and one of the study's authors. "High glucose in diabetes leaves trace chemicals harmful to cells—that process is called oxidative stress." Oxidative stress is implicated in many disease processes, including diabetic neuropathy, he says. "If you burn something in the oven, it leaves soot. Similarly, in disease, there is 'soot,' and there are mechanisms that relieve 'soot.' Antioxidants promote getting rid of oxidative stress products."

■ **WHAT TO TAKE/DOSAGES:** Studies that have examined the potential benefits of ALA and neuropathy suggest that 600 to 1,200 milligrams a day is needed to gain the benefits.

Calcium and Vitamin D in Combination

■ **WHAT IT IS:** The mineral calcium helps keep your bones hard and strong. Vitamin D, which the body makes when the skin is exposed to sunlight, helps the body absorb calcium. Both of these nutrients are important to good health. However, recent research suggests that double-teaming them can provide benefits that go beyond stronger bones.

■ **WHAT WE KNOW:** Calcium plus vitamin D offers powerful protection against diabetes, a landmark study suggests. In a 20-year study of 83,779 women by scientists at Tufts–New England Medical Center in Boston, those who were getting the highest levels of the combo—more than 1,200 milligrams of calcium and more than 800 IU of D daily—had a 33 percent lower risk of type 2 diabetes than women who were getting the lowest dose. The nutrients also worked alone, though not as well. About 75 percent of the women got less than the recommended levels of calcium, and 97 percent got too little D. That's not surprising. "Vitamin D deficiency is common in the general population and perhaps more common in people with diabetes," says Dr. Bradley.

■ **WHAT TO TAKE/DOSAGES:** Take a 500-milligram supplement of calcium daily (unless you're at risk for brittle bones), and add a D pill containing 400 IU. Aim for one to two servings of low-fat dairy, too.

Chromium

■ **WHAT IT IS:** This mineral helps the body metabolize and store carbohydrate, protein, and fat and is known to enhance the action of insulin. A deficiency in chromium impairs the body's ability to use glucose, thereby increasing its need for insulin.

■ **WHAT WE KNOW:** Studies designed to test chromium's effect on blood sugar have yielded mixed results. Part of the problem: Each study used different dosages or formulations of chromium, and several of the studies were poorly designed. Lacking solid evidence from good clinical trials, the American Diabetes Association does not recommend chromium supplementation.

However, one recent well-designed clinical trial *has* shown benefit, says Dr. Bradley. In a 2006 study, researchers led by Julie Martin, RD, of the University of Vermont investigated chromium supplementation in 39 people with diabetes who also took the medication glipizide (Glucotrol). The volunteers took 1,000 micrograms of chromium picolinate for 24 weeks. At the end of the study, "those who took chromium had an average hemoglobin A1C reduction of 1.13 percent, improved insulin sensitivity, and [showed] an improvement in

SELENIUM SUPPLEMENTS: DON'T HELP, MAY HURT

Selenium supplements do appear to affect the risk of type 2 diabetes—but not the way researchers had hoped. Rather than help fend off the disease, extra doses of the mineral (found in soil and some foods) may instead contribute to its development.

A team of British and American researchers wanted to find out if selenium—found to help control blood sugar and delay complications of diabetes in animal studies—might help prevent diabetes in humans. So they collected data on 1,202 people in the United States with skin cancer who were enrolled in a study designed primarily to test selenium's ability to help prevent cancer. All of the study's subjects lived in areas with low levels of selenium in the soil, and none reported having type 2 diabetes.

The researchers measured the level of selenium in the volunteers' blood, then divided them into two groups. One group received a daily 200-microgram selenium supplement; the other got a placebo. After 8 years, the researchers found that the risk of developing diabetes was about 50 percent higher among those in the selenium group, compared with those taking a placebo.

"The hypothesis was that, because of its antioxidant properties, selenium could be beneficial in diabetes prevention," says lead researcher Saverio Stranges, MD. "In fact, long-term selenium supplementation did not have any benefits in diabetes prevention and actually increased the risk for this disease."

An editorial that accompanied the study said that although the primary causes of diabetes are obesity and lack of physical activity, "environmental exposures may also be important." The editorial noted, too, that most people in the United States get enough selenium through diet alone. "By taking selenium supplements on top of an adequate dietary intake, people may increase their risk for diabetes," the editorial stated.

This single study doesn't prove that selenium increases the risk for diabetes, says Eliseo Guallar, MD, of Johns Hopkins University Bloomberg School of Public Health, a coauthor of the editorial. "But it's enough to say this is worrisome," he says. "Until we know for sure that there are benefits from these supplements, it doesn't make sense to take them."

their percent of body fat," says Dr. Bradley. "Since glipizide is a first-line oral medication for the treatment of diabetes, studying chromium with this medication has significant clinical value."

Some conventional medicine practitioners recommend chromium supplementation, too. "Although the FDA has not endorsed chromium's role in insulin resistance, I have found it quite valuable in patients with metabolic syndrome, insulin resistance, and significant carbohydrate cravings, likely due to the essential role chromium plays in the function of insulin," says Melina Jampolis, MD, a San Francisco–based physician and author of *The No Time to Lose Diet*. "In my practice, it leads to a clinically significant reduction in blood sugar."

■ **WHAT TO TAKE/DOSAGES:** Chromium is available in a variety of forms: as a single supplement, as an ingredient in multivitamins, or combined with any number of vitamins and/or minerals. Chromium picolinate and chromium histidine are believed to be better absorbed than other forms of the mineral.

Dr. Jampolis suggests that her diabetes patients try Glucoset, which contains chromium, the B-complex vitamin biotin, ALA, and gymnema sylvestre. "They all play a role in the utilization of blood sugar metabolism and insulin action," she says. Dr. Bradley suggests Diachrome, which teams chromium picolinate with biotin. Regardless of which brand you select, follow the dosage instructions on the label.

Cinnamon

■ **WHAT IT IS:** We use this fragrant spice—actually, the dried bark of a small evergreen tree cultivated throughout Asia—to flavor apple pie and other goodies. However, ancient healers in China, Greece, and India viewed cinnamon as medicine, using it to treat maladies from kidney disorders to digestive problems.

■ **WHAT WE KNOW:** A number of clinical studies have shown that cinnamon can lower cholesterol and triglycerides and rein in blood sugar. "The data on cinnamon is unquestionable," says Dr. Jampolis.

For example, researchers from the Beltsville Human Nutrition Research Center in Maryland, part of the USDA, reported on a study of 60 people with type 2 diabetes in Pakistan. The 40-day study found that 1 gram of cinnamon a day—that's $\frac{1}{4}$ teaspoon twice a day—lowered blood sugar by an average of 18 to 29 percent, triglycerides (fatty acids in the blood) by 23 to 30 percent, "bad" LDL cholesterol by 7 to 27 percent, and total cholesterol by 12 to 26 percent. It's thought that natural plant chemicals called polyphenols may activate enzymes that stimulate insulin receptors.

■ **WHAT TO TAKE/DOSAGES:** Dosages of 1 to 6 grams a day were used in studies (1 gram equals about $\frac{1}{2}$ teaspoon. Typical recommendations are 1 to 3 grams a day of a water-based cinnamon extract, which is used in brands such as CinnaBeticII and Cinnulin PF.

Fenugreek

■ **WHAT IT IS:** If you enjoy Indian curry, you've tasted this spice, made from the dried seeds of *Trigonella foenum-graecum*. In ancient Egypt, extracts of the herb were used to embalm mummies; in ancient Rome, to aid in labor and delivery. In traditional Chinese medicine, the seeds are used as a tonic.

■ **WHAT WE KNOW:** Fenugreek seeds are high in soluble fiber, which slows carbohydrate digestion and absorption, thereby delaying the rise of blood sugar. Animal research suggests that fenugreek may also contain a substance that stimulates insulin production and improves blood sugar control. Plant chemicals called saponins in the seeds may be responsible for fenugreek's ability to lower triglycerides, LDL cholesterol, and total cholesterol.

A few small studies have found that fenugreek may help lower blood sugar levels in people with diabetes. In one study, researchers from India divided 25 people newly diagnosed with type 2 diabetes into two groups. The first group received fenugreek (1 gram per day of a standardized extract). The second group was given a placebo. After 2 months, the researchers found that the fenugreek group had significant improvements on some measures of blood

GET SAVVY ABOUT SUPPLEMENTS

In 2005, the FDA issued a nationwide alert against Liqiang 4, a supplement made in China promoted as useful for diabetes management. Marketed as "all-natural," Liqiang 4 was far from it. This supplement contained glyburide, a prescription drug used to treat type 2 diabetes.

In FDA-approved medications, glyburide is safe. However, people with type 2 diabetes who took Liqiang 4 could receive dangerously high amounts. Thankfully, no deaths were reported.

The case of Liqiang 4 was nothing new. In the past, supplements have been recalled because they were found to be contaminated with microbes, pesticides, and heavy metals or because they contained more or less than the amount of the dietary ingredient on the label.

In 2007, the FDA passed new laws governing supplements. They require manufacturers to meet tougher standards to show that their products are safe and contain exactly what the label says. However, these regulations won't apply to all manufacturers until 2010. In the meantime, the tips below can help ensure the supplements you buy are safe and effective.

- Select supplements manufactured by national food and supplement companies. Check the expiration date, too.

- Pass on foreign supplements, especially those made in China and India. They're more likely to contain dangerous contaminants.

- Select supplements made with standardized extracts. The label should clearly identify the quantities of the active ingredients.

- Look for supplements that have recognized symbols of quality, such as the USP, NF, TruLabel, or ConsumerLab symbol.

sugar control and insulin response. Their triglyceride levels fell and their "good" HDL cholesterol rose significantly, too—presumably due to the enhanced insulin sensitivity. In another study, taking 2.5 grams of fenugreek twice a day for 3 months reduced blood sugar levels in people with mild (but not those with severe) type 2 diabetes.

■ **WHAT TO TAKE/DOSAGES:** Fenugreek seeds tend to have a bitter taste, so most people prefer debitterized seeds or capsules. The typical range of intake for diabetes or to lower cholesterol is 5 to 30 grams (1 teaspoon to about 2½ tablespoons) with each meal or 15 to 90 grams all at once with one meal. As a tincture, 3 to 4 milliliters of fenugreek can be taken up to three times per day.

Fish Oils

■ **WHAT THEY ARE:** Oil from fatty fish like mackerel, lake trout, herring, sardines, albacore tuna, and salmon contains eicosapentaenoic acid (EPA) and docosahexaenoic acid (DHA). Both are omega-3 fatty acids.

■ **WHAT WE KNOW:** Omega-3 fatty acids benefit the hearts of people at high risk for heart disease or those who already have it. These oily marvels protect the heart's natural rhythm, guarding against the sudden uncoordinated heartbeats that can cause death during a heart attack. Randomized clinical trials have shown that omega-3 fatty acid supplements can slow the progression of atherosclerosis in people with heart disease, as well as reduce the incidence of nonfatal heart attacks and strokes.

In studies of 773 people, researchers from the University of Washington, Seattle, and the University of Kuopio in Finland found that those with the highest blood levels of EPA and DHA had a 50 to 65 percent lower risk of fatal heart attack or stroke than those with the lowest levels. Fish oil also seems to safely and effectively reduce triglyceride levels in people with diabetes.

■ **WHAT TO TAKE/DOSAGES:** Evidence suggests that taking from 0.5 to 1.8 grams of EPA and DHA per day, either as fatty fish or supplements, significantly reduces deaths from heart disease. If you have diabetes and heart disease or high triglycerides, ask your doctor if taking EPA and DHA in capsule form is right for you. The American Heart Association recommends taking 1 gram per day for people with heart disease and 2 to 4 grams a day for people with high triglycerides—under a doctor's supervision.

Ginseng, American

■ **WHAT IT IS:** Ginseng is derived from the root of the *Panax* genus of plants. There are different species of this herb, including Asian ginseng (*Panax ginseng*), American ginseng (*Panax quinquefolius*), and Siberian ginseng (*Eleutherococcus senticosus*). All have been advocated to boost immune function and treat a variety of conditions from fatigue to cancer. Studies of ginseng's effects on diabetes primarily have used American ginseng.

■ **WHAT WE KNOW:** Clinical trials of American ginseng in people with type 2 diabetes have shown reductions in hemoglobin A1C and fasting blood sugar. This herb also has proven effective in reducing high blood sugar after a meal.

In a small pilot study, researchers gave nine people with type 2 diabetes either 3 grams of American ginseng or placebo capsules, either 40 minutes before or together with a high-glucose drink. Their blood sugar declined significantly, whether they took the ginseng before or with the drink. In a follow-up study, American ginseng controlled the rise in blood sugar up to 2 hours before the beverage did.

Most of ginseng's health benefits are attributed to natural plant chemicals called ginsenosides, which researchers believe stimulate cells in the pancreas to make more insulin. American ginseng may also help remove glucose from the blood and slow its absorption from food.

■ **WHAT TO TAKE/DOSAGES:** Ginseng comes in different forms, including the raw root, capsules, tablets, and extracts. The typical recommended daily dosage of *Panax ginseng* is 1 to 2 grams of raw herb (¼ to ½ teaspoon) or 200 milligrams daily of a capsule, tablet, or extract standardized containing 4 to 7 percent ginsenosides. One study of American ginseng for diabetes used 3 grams daily.

Gymnema

■ **WHAT IT IS:** For more than 2,000 years, people have chewed the leaves of this woody plant, which grows in the tropical forests of India and Africa, to treat *madhu meha,* or "honey urine." "Gymnema is known as 'sugar destroyer' in Ayurvedic healing traditions," says Dr. Bradley.

■ **WHAT WE KNOW:** Gymnema increases the activity of enzymes responsible for taking up and using blood sugar. It also may stimulate the pancreas to produce insulin or increase the release of insulin.

"Clinical trials of gymnema in diabetes are limited, but two existing trials do demonstrate positive effects," says Dr. Bradley. In one preliminary study of people with type 2 diabetes, researchers reported that 400 milligrams per day of gymnema extract taken for periods of 18 months or longer resulted in improvement in blood sugar levels, according to blood tests, and allowed reduction of diabetes medications. In fact, 5 of the 22 participants were able to discontinue their conventional medications during the trial. Another preliminary trial found improved blood sugar levels after 3 months in a group of people with both type 1 and type 2 diabetes who took 800 milligrams per day of a gymnema extract standardized for 25 percent gymnemic acids.

■ **WHAT TO TAKE/DOSAGES:** Typically, dosage is 400 to 600 milligrams daily of an extract standardized to contain 25 percent gymnemic acids.

Magnesium

■ **WHAT IT IS:** Used in more than 300 biochemical reactions in the body, magnesium helps keep bones strong, the heartbeat steady, and muscles and nerves functioning normally. This mineral also plays an important role in carbohydrate metabolism. It helps regulate blood sugar levels and may influence the release and activity of insulin.

■ **WHAT WE KNOW:** As many as one out of every three people with diabetes is low on this mineral. What's more, research shows that as magnesium intake goes up, the risk of developing type 2 diabetes goes down.

Several studies have examined the potential benefit of supplemental magnesium on control of type 2 diabetes. In one study, researchers in Mexico gave 63 people with type 2 diabetes and below-normal blood levels of magnesium either 2.5 grams of magnesium a day (in a liquid form that provided 300 mil-

EGCG: NEW HELP FOR DIABETES ON THE HORIZON?

Research links drinking several cups of green tea a day with a lower risk of type 2 diabetes, thanks to a compound called epigallocatechin gallate. Might EGCG supplements help lower diabetes risk as well?

More study is needed. But in tests on mice with diabetes, EGCG extract worked as well as the diabetes drug rosiglitazone (Avandia). (Note: In May 2007, the FDA slapped Avandia with a black box label indicating the potential for life-threatening side effects.) That's according to researchers from the Karolinska Institute in Sweden, who fed moderately and severely diabetic mice either EGCG extract or rosiglitazone. Their blood sugar and insulin levels were studied after 5 and 10 weeks of treatment. While mice with severe diabetes did not benefit as much from EGCG, those with moderate diabetes did as well on EGCG as on rosiglitazone.

The researchers said that EGCG preserved insulin-producing tissue in the mice's pancreases and limited damage that could worsen diabetes. This suggests that green tea extract supplements may also help treat diabetes in humans.

ligrams magnesium per day) or a placebo. At the end of the 16-week study, the researchers found that, compared with those who had received a placebo, those who'd taken the magnesium had higher levels of magnesium in their blood. Their insulin sensitivity and metabolic control of their diabetes also improved, as suggested by their lower levels of hemoglobin A1C.

■ **WHAT TO TAKE/DOSAGES:** Many doctors recommend that people with diabetes and normal kidney function supplement with 200 to 600 milligrams of magnesium per day. You can find supplements in a variety of forms. One study found magnesium citrate to be well absorbed.

9. Make Exercise an Everyday Event

"EXERCISE IS LIKE BRUSHING YOUR TEETH. When we were little, our parents always encouraged us to brush our teeth, and that was the last thing we wanted to do. Then one day we went to the dentist and had a cavity," says Jennifer Hopper, an exercise physiologist at Piedmont Hospital in Atlanta, who frequently works with patients with newly diagnosed diabetes.

To teach clients about the importance of exercise, she asks them to think a moment about their teeth. "The dentist told us, 'If you begin to brush your teeth regularly, this will prevent any more cavities from occurring.' I tell patients, 'This diagnosis is your cavity, and exercise is going to be the preventive action, like brushing your teeth, to help you manage this. It's time for you to take control of your body.'"

Dentists may encourage their patients to brush—or floss, an unappealing chore for many—by urging them to find ways to make it easier. Instead of making yourself floss at the end of the day when you just want to get to bed, do it while you're watching TV! Similarly, experts in diabetes and exercise encourage you to see this practice more as "physical activity" and find ways to fit it painlessly into your day. If necessary, do it in little chunks instead of 30-minute blocks—do it while you're watching TV!

However you do it, just be sure that you do it.

Little Increments Really Add Up

The American Diabetes Association (ADA) recommends that people with type 2 diabetes get at least 150 minutes of moderate aerobic physical activity each week or at least 90 minutes of vigorous activity. This is enough to help you improve blood sugar control, lose weight or keep it off, and lower your risk of heart disease.

You should spread out this total time over at least 3 days, and don't go more than 2 consecutive days without physical activity. A single bout of exercise can make your body less resistant to its insulin for 24 to 72 hours, so you want to keep recharging yourself with frequent activity to hang on to this effect.

If you have prediabetes, exercise is important to keep it from turning into diabetes. Research has found that exercising for 30 minutes most days of the week, as part of a program to lose 5 to 7 percent of your body weight if you're overweight, is a crucial part of avoiding or delaying type 2 diabetes.

If you can find the time and motivation to work out for 30 minutes straight, that's great. (See "Move a Little, Gain a Lot" on page 316 for some ideas.) Otherwise, fit in physical activity wherever you can.

"What I've ended up advocating more than anything for people with diabetes, especially for type 2, is to fit exercise into the day in an unstructured way whenever and wherever possible. You don't realize how much of an impact that has," says Sheri Colberg, PhD, an author, professor, and exercise physiologist who has diabetes. "If you're going to do your 30 minutes of structured exercise in a day, you'll expend more calories at a faster rate," she says. "But then you've got 23½ other hours in the day; and in those other 23½ hours, you can do all kinds of things that expend energy and work your muscles."

In one study, researchers found that normal-weight people stood up for 2½ hours a day more than overweight people did, Dr. Colberg says. "I know the author of that study, and whenever he goes to lectures, he stands up in the back of the lecture hall," she adds.

Gary Scheiner, CDE, a Wynnewood, Pennsylvania, exercise physiologist and diabetes educator who's had diabetes for several decades, echoes the message of not always associating physical activity with putting on workout clothes, driving to the gym, and sweating for 30 minutes. It can mean rein-

MOVE A LITTLE, GAIN A LOT

Getting your body moving is as simple as, well, getting up and moving. Here are a few creative ways to sneak more physical activity into your day. In general, try to do things the old-fashioned way: Take care of chores by hand instead of using modern conveniences designed to take the work away.

- Use a push mower instead of a riding mower.

- Use a rake instead of a leaf blower.

- Plant a garden—all that digging, weeding, and picking provides exercise throughout the spring and summer.

- Stand up and walk around while you're using the phone.

- Consult with co-workers in person instead of using the phone or e-mail.

- Whenever you're waiting—for your plane to take off, a restaurant table to open up—stand up and walk around instead of sitting.

- Take active vacations. Seek out guided walking or biking tours of a city, go hiking, or walk on the beach.

- If you're a parent (or grandparent), participate in playtime instead of just watching the kids run around. If you have a pet, take it for a walk instead of letting it outside alone.

- Carry a basket instead of pushing a cart at the grocery store.

- Stir foods with a whisk or long-handled spoon instead of an electric mixer. Open cans with a manual can opener instead of an electric one.

- Keep a timer by your television or computer and set it to ring after 30 minutes. That's your signal to get up and move around.

serting some of the everyday effort that our modern world has taken away from simple tasks.

"You can't even go to the bathroom anymore without an automatic thing feeding you toilet paper, and you don't even turn the handle on the faucet. There's no physical movement involved in a lot of things we do anymore. We're sitting, sitting, sitting, and we're not moving enough," Scheiner says. "A lot of the changes we try to get people to make are simple things, using fewer convenience devices and getting up and moving more."

Likewise, if you're overweight and underactive—which is the story for many people with type 2 diabetes or prediabetes—it's okay to ease into exercise, Dr. Colberg and Scheiner say. If you can walk only a few minutes at a time at first, that's fine—just walk a few minutes. Very slowly add a bit more from week to week, and keep incorporating more physical movement into your life.

"I never want exercise to be painful to people. It should feel good," Scheiner says. "I like people to succeed up front. If you set people up to succeed, it's going to work. If you set them up to fail, it's going to fail. For most people, it took 20, 30, or 40 years to get into the shape they're currently in, and you can't expect to reverse that in a week or two. It's going to take time."

In Dr. Colberg's experience, "once people start to feel a little bit better, they're standing more and walking a little bit more; they have more energy. They didn't realize how bad they felt before they started doing that. Once they have more energy, then maybe it's going to be easier to start that structured program. They realize that's not so hard—maybe they can do 15 or 20 minutes."

Although aerobic exercise is important, it represents only part of your weekly activity needs—you need to strengthen your muscles, too. As we discussed earlier in this book, your muscles start dwindling after age 30, and the decline really gains speed after 60, setting the stage for weight gain and insulin resistance. The antidote: strength-training, which will help you preserve your muscles. The ADA urges you to do resistance exercise three times a week. You can lift weights, tug against elastic resistance bands, or use weight machines.

JUST A FEW EXERCISES
WILL DO A BODY GOOD

Need a basic strength-training program? Try these moves recommended by experts. Start with light weights and few repetitions, gradually increasing to heavier weights and 8 to 10 repetitions as your strength improves.

- Chest press: Lie on your back on a bench, holding a pair of dumbells or a bar-bell. Raise the weight straight toward the ceiling over your chest, pause a moment, then lower to the starting position. Repeat.

- Biceps curls: While standing, hold a dumbbell in one hand, palm facing out. Let your arm hang down at thigh level. Now slowly lift the weight toward your shoulder. Lower and repeat, then switch hands.

- Triceps extension: Lie on your back on a bench, holding a dumbell in one hand. Bend your elbow so that the weight is at your shoulder. Raise the weight straight toward the ceiling, then slowly lower it back toward your shoulder. Your elbow should stay stationary and pointed toward the ceiling. Repeat, then switch hands.

- Bent-over row: Lean over a bench, bracing yourself with one knee and one hand. Hold a dumbbell in your free hand, with your arm hanging toward the floor. Draw your elbow back so that the weight comes to the side of your chest. Pause, lower the weight to the starting position, and repeat. Then switch hands.

- Knee extension: Sitting on a bench with an ankle weight on one foot, raise your leg in front of you until it's horizontal with the floor. Slowly lower the weight and repeat, then switch legs.

- Curl-ups: Lie on your back on the floor with one knee bent and your foot flat on the floor. Extend the other leg. Keeping your arms crossed over your chest, lift your upper body off the floor a few inches. Pause a moment, slowly lower your-self, and repeat. Then switch legs.

- Back extension: Lie facedown on the floor with your legs fully extended and your arms at your sides. Lift your upper body off the floor a few inches, using your lower back muscles. Hold a moment, then slowly lower your upper body and repeat.

Choosing the Right Exercise for You

Many fitness authorities recommend walking as a simple, inexpensive activity for people who have diabetes. But even this exercise isn't always ideal. "We try to get people to walk," says Kristi Holden, an exercise physiologist at Gritman Medical Center in Moscow, Idaho, who regularly helps steer people with diabetes into an exercise program. The problem: "Around here, they say, 'I'm going to start this great walking program, and I have it all mapped out.' Then it snows, and they say, 'Oh, I don't feel like walking today.' And in the summer it can get over 100 degrees."

The lessons here: First, even if you love a particular activity, have others that you can fall back on. If you enjoy hiking around the hills in your neighborhood, be willing to walk around the mall on rainy days. If you play racquetball with a friend three times a week, be ready for a solo sport on days your pal can't make it. Second, engaging in a variety of activities prevents any one from growing stale, Holden says. If you go to a health club, rotate your workouts between the treadmill, elliptical trainer, and other cardio machines. Boredom is a common reason for not heading to the gym, so try to nip that excuse before it even buds.

If you're having trouble coming up with appealing types of exercise, think about what sorts of activities interest you, Scheiner suggests. Different activities tap into different desires that can provide motivation. For example:

DO YOU LIKE SOLITUDE? Perhaps using exercise tapes at home or walking on trails in a nearby state park would inspire you.

■ **DO YOU LIKE COMPANY?** Taking exercise classes at a gym offers a good way to meet people. Less expensive alternatives: Join a walking club or organization that's training for an upcoming road race, or sign up for a team sport at your workplace.

■ **IS MONEY A PROBLEM?** "It doesn't cost a penny to exercise," Hopper says. Walking is free, and so is dancing or raking leaves. For strength-training, just get on the floor and do crunches and push-ups. Too hard? Do push-ups against a wall.

■ **DO YOU LIKE NUMBERS OR GADGETS?** You can track your progress on stairclimbers, treadmills, and other gym equipment that shows you your elapsed time, calories expended, and miles covered. Jot down your results in a notebook. If you like gadgets and gear, you can pick up all sorts of cool equipment for running and biking, such as a heart-rate monitor and a wristwatch with a GPS tracking feature.

Not every type of workout is appropriate for people with diabetes because the disease puts you at higher risk for eye and foot damage, and you don't want to further injure yourself with exercise, Scheiner says. If you have problems with your feet, such as numbness and poor circulation, even walking may not be wise. Cycling, swimming, rowing, or water aerobics may be foot-friendlier choices, says Scheiner. If you have damage to your retinas (the lining in your eyes), it may be a bad idea to engage in exercise that's jarring or requires you to strain, such as lifting weights, martial arts, jogging, high-impact aerobics, or racquet sports.

However, avoiding certain moves doesn't mean avoiding all movement. "There's no reason that people can't find something they can do. There are always options," Scheiner says. "I don't want people to think that just because they're in horrible shape or have all these illnesses, there's nothing they can do. There's always something if they look for it."

Make It Fun and Get It Done

Physical activity should be doable and gratifying—not a huge challenge that you have to struggle to master, Hopper says. If it feels like a burden, you won't stick with it. It shouldn't cause discomfort and certainly not pain. At the end of a session, you should feel like you could have done a little more, as though you have energy left over for your next round. Here are some of the experts' recommendations to get physical in your daily life.

■ **EASE INTO IT.** If you're new to physical activity, you'll end up with sore muscles if you push your body too much the first time or two. If you can walk

GET CHARGED UP BEFORE YOU START

Kristi Holden, an exercise physiologist at Gritman Medical Center in Moscow, Idaho, often works with people with diabetes. She makes sure they're aware of the following recommendations from the American Diabetes Association for preventing low blood sugar while exercising.

First test your blood sugar. Then . . .

For light exercise (a walk or bike ride of less than 30 minutes):

- If your blood sugar is less than 80, eat 5 to 8 grams of carbohydrate per hour.

- If it's 80 to 100, consider eating 10 to 15 grams of carbohydrate before your session.

For moderate exercise (such as jogging or playing tennis):

- If your blood sugar is less than 80, eat 25 to 35 grams of carbohydrate before leaving, then 10 to 15 grams for each half-hour of exercise.

- If your blood sugar is 80 to 180, eat 10 to 15 grams per half-hour of exercise.

For a strenuous workout:

- If your blood sugar is under 80, eat about 50 grams of carbohydrate, perhaps also with a source of protein or fat.

- If your blood sugar is 80 to 180, eat 25 to 50 grams of carbohydrate.

Good sources of carbohydrate before exercise include fruit, juice, fat-free milk, and bread.

---

only 10 minutes or 5 minutes or even less at first, that's fine. Don't go for a full half-hour if your body isn't ready for the challenge.

■ **GET A PEDOMETER.** These step-counting devices are cheap and easily found at department stores. Clip one to your waist and see how many steps you take in an average day, Scheiner recommends. Try to tally more steps next week; whether it's another 100 or 1,000 is up to you—just keep the goal small and attainable.

■ **INK IT IN.** At the beginning of each week, plot when you're going to get your structured exercise, Dr. Colberg recommends. Block it out on your desk calendar or electronic organizer. This is a lifesaving appointment, so don't let meetings or other time-stealers keep you from it, she urges.

■ **MAKE IT MODERATE.** "Moderate exercise is the way to go," Holden says. If you're gasping and panting, you're going at it harder than you have to do. Here's a simple way to judge your pace: If you could deliver a speech while you're exercising, notch up a bit. If you couldn't speak more than a few words to someone, bring it down. If you could carry on a conversation, with a few pauses for breath, you're on a moderate target.

■ **PAL AROUND.** Having an exercise buddy or attending an exercise class keeps you motivated—it's fun to socialize, and other people count on you to show up, Holden says. Best of all, enlist your significant other—the partner of someone with diabetes is at added risk for developing the condition, too.

■ **TIME IT RIGHT.** Some people find a morning workout exhilarating—but not everyone. "I could never exercise in the morning. I'd be so relaxed I'd be drooling on myself by noon," says Hopper. If a morning walk would wear you out, do it in the evening instead.

■ **BE CONSISTENT.** Remember, you only get the benefits of exercise if you actually do it. As we mentioned earlier, the improvements in your insulin resistance last only so long—no more than 72 hours—so you have to keep lacing up your shoes regularly. This is a long-term commitment, Hopper says. Keep your goals small, and very gradually increase your length or intensity of activity over weeks and months so you'll stay motivated to continue.

Head Off Hypoglycemia

The general goal in diabetes is to keep your blood sugar from rising too high. But when you're physically active, you need to pay attention to keep your blood sugar from getting too *low*. Because exercise causes your blood sugar to drop, you may be more prone to develop hypoglycemia, an episode of too-low blood sugar that can be dangerous—particularly if you're walking, biking, or doing other activities away from home, Holden says. You're more prone to hypoglycemia during exercise if you're taking insulin or a sulfonylurea drug to control blood sugar, Scheiner says. To reduce your risk:

- Follow a schedule. Your blood sugar will respond differently to exercise at different times of day, partly because the amount of time between your meals varies, Holden says. Try to do extended sessions at the same time from day to day so your blood sugar will respond reliably.

- Visit an exercise physiologist. One of these professionals—particularly one with an interest in diabetes—can help you plan your activities, set goals, and ward off injury, Scheiner says. Check out the American Association of Diabetes Educators at diabeteseducator.org or the Diabetes Exercise and Sports Association at diabetes-exercise.org/index.asp to look for an exercise pro in your area.

- Check your blood sugar first. Before you stick your feet into your workout shoes, stick a lancet into your finger and check your blood sugar, Holden recommends. This is particularly important information when you're just starting an exercise program. If your blood sugar is too low, you should eat a snack before starting a workout. Or if you use medications, cut back before exercise after consulting with your doctor—if you're trying to shed pounds, this may be a better strategy than snacking more, Scheiner says.

- Watch where you poke. You'll absorb insulin more quickly if you inject it over a working muscle. If you're going to exercise within 30 minutes, inject near a muscle that won't be doing much work—so if you're walking, avoid the legs.

- Know when to skip it. If your blood sugar is more than 300, don't exercise because it could make your levels rise further. If it's more than 240 and a test shows that your urine contains ketones, don't exercise then, either.

SHOE SHOPPING POINTERS

When it comes to walking workouts, there's nothing more important than a good shoe. "Don't think that you can just go to the store and pick out cheap fitness shoes simply because you are a beginner or don't walk much," says Melinda Reiner, DPM, vice president of the American Association for Women Podiatrists. Different feet need different shoes. To find a perfect pair, keep these tips in mind.

Choose walking shoes. Any old shoe may work, but one designed for walking will decrease your risk of injury and boost performance. A good one will be flexible in the ball of the foot but not the arch. (A shoe that bends in the arch will place increased stress on the plantar fascia.) The heel should be cushioned (you don't need a lot of padding in the forefoot) and rounded to speed your foot through the heel-toe motion with ease.

Go offline for a fit. This is one purchase that must be made in person. Whether you have low arches or tend to overpronate, the salespeople in a good technical running store will watch you walk barefoot and help you choose the features you need. Best to try: a store that's independently owned.

Buy big. Women especially tend to buy shoes that are too small. Ask the salesperson to help you check the fit, and don't get caught up in thinking that you have to buy a size 8 because that's what you've always worn. Athletic shoes can be sized quite differently from your dress shoes.

Toss 'em often. Don't skimp on your feet. Once the interior padding has lost its spring, it's time for a new pair. Generally, that means replacing your shoes every 500 miles—sooner if you have foot, ankle, knee, or back problems.

■ Drink plenty. Dehydration can affect your blood sugar. Drink 16 ounces of fluid 2 hours before exercise and down plenty more during the workout—especially if it's hot outdoors.

- Know the signs of trouble. If you feel shaky, anxious, or hungry, or your heartbeat changes or you start sweating more, you might have hypoglycemia. Carry candy or juice so you can help bring your blood sugar back up. Before you begin exercising, ask your doctor how to address this issue.

Diabetes Rx

Whatever exercise you choose, here are the general guidelines for managing your blood sugar, getting fit—and staying safe.

- Get at least 150 minutes of moderate aerobic activity each week, divided among at least 3 days.

- Ease into exercise slowly. If you can't do half an hour at a time, break it up into smaller bouts throughout the day. When you *are* doing 30-minute sessions, incorporate more movement into everyday activities.

- Strength-train three times a week, choosing exercises that work all your major muscle groups. Work your way up until you're doing three sets of 8 to 10 repetitions per move. Use a weight at which the last couple of reps are difficult but can still be done using proper form.

- Do a variety of activities; known as cross-training, this ensures you work different muscles at different times and keep your body challenged. Plus, you won't get bored, and you'll have options on days you can't do your favorite activity.

- Wear good-fitting, comfortable shoes and socks, and check your feet for blisters and other injuries before and after exercise.

- Check your blood sugar before you start an exercise session. Take precautions to avoid hypoglycemia, such as eating carbohydrates before beginning and carrying rescue foods such as hard candy.

- Visit your doctor before starting an exercise program or increasing your physical activity. Describe the details of your plan, such as what activities you're going to do, how often, and how vigorously. Your doctor should examine you—and perhaps order tests—to ensure that your heart is healthy enough for extra demands, your eyes can handle the movements, and your feet are in shape for the challenge. If there are any concerns, your doctor should help you design a program that will minimize the risk of injury.

- Keep a cell phone with you, carry ID, and wear a bracelet or other form of notification that you have diabetes.

10. Adopt a Positive "Diatitude"

IN COLUMBUS, GEORGIA, you'll find a medical practice focusing on diabetes and other hormonal disorders, where patients can work with four endocrinologists, a nurse educator, and a dietitian.

If a patient's A1C levels—a measure of long-term blood sugar control—remain too high despite everyone's efforts, he or she is referred to one other provider on staff: Elizabeth Dreelin, PhD, a clinical psychologist who focuses on diabetes issues. She not only helps patients deal with stress and depression—which, as we discussed earlier, can have a major impact on diabetes control—she also helps them develop healthy behaviors and attitudes regarding the disease.

Diabetes Rx

By applying a positive attitude to your diabetes—let's call it your diatitude—you can keep your mind calm and your body better protected from this disease. Here are some of Dr. Dreelin's and other experts' top recommendations for creating a positive diatitude.

▪ **GET INFORMED.** To reduce stress related to your diabetes, educate yourself about the disease, says Mary Ann Koch, PhD, a Roanoke, Virginia, psychologist who has counseled many patients with diabetes over the past 2 decades. When you're uninformed or harboring untrue beliefs about diabetes, the condition may seem much scarier than it does when you're armed with the facts.

If you're confused about a diabetes issue, write down your questions for your doctor or diabetes educator so you remember to ask them at your next opportunity. If diabetes education classes are available in your area, go to them. Visit reputable diabetes Web sites, such as the American Diabetes Association (diabetes.org) or the National Institutes of Health's diabetes section (diabetes.niddk.nih.gov/). Be sure your family members become educated about this disease, too, Dr. Koch suggests. This will put them in a better position to help you and will also help alleviate some of the worries that they might have.

■ **GET SUPPORT.** Seek out other people who are resolving their diabetes challenges in a positive manner, Dr. Koch recommends—maybe a friend, perhaps a support group that meets online or in person. When you discuss your problems with someone who understands them well, you might learn creative new solutions that others have discovered. Contact your local hospital to see if a support group meets in your area, or log on to an online group at the ADA Web site or the diabetes Web site dLife.com.

■ **EXERCISE.** One of the simplest ways to reduce depression and stress is free . . . and it's something you should be doing anyway to control your blood sugar: Get your body moving.

"There's now enough evidence to really recommend exercise as part of standard treatment of depression. Good studies show that regular aerobic exercise—and I don't mean every day for an hour, but 20 minutes three times a week—can have as much effect on depression as an SSRI [a type of antidepressant] such as Zoloft," says Susan Guzman, PhD, head of adult clinical services at the Behavioral Diabetes Institute in San Diego.

Aside from providing a psychological lift, exercise also lowers your blood sugar, which in turn makes you feel less groggy and depressed, Dr. Dreelin says. She suggests that in addition to activities such as walking, cycling, water aerobics, and strength-training, you consider yoga. It relieves muscle tension, encourages you to breathe deeply, relaxes you, and improves sleep.

■ **MAKE SELF-CARE A PRIORITY.** When you're stressed, it's especially important to protect your mental and physical health . . . but ironically, that's "often the last thing we do," Dr. Guzman says. No matter how frazzled you feel, make time for exercise and stress relief. Not only is exercise good for depression, it also helps your body better cope with the physical effects of stress, she says. Set an alarm, and when it goes off, take a moment to do a session of progressive muscle relaxation. Or set an appointment on your computer's calendar to remind you to take a break at noon for a healthy lunch and a walk. Make these stress-busters a priority in your schedule.

■ **CHANGE YOUR THOUGHTS AND BEHAVIORS.** In the chapter on stress (page 262), you learned about an effective approach called cognitive-behavioral therapy. This requires that you examine the thoughts and behaviors that are contributing to your stress and exchange them for healthier ways of thinking and acting. These steps will help reduce your depression, Dr. Guzman says, who uses this approach with her clients, both in individual and group counseling, to challenge their distorted ways of thinking and to turn around their negative beliefs. But you can use cognitive-behavioral steps on your own. Here are a few ways to get your diabetes-related thoughts and actions on a new track.

■ Avoid all-or-nothing thinking. People with depression often see their behaviors in a way that requires perfection. "If you eat a piece of cake you didn't really need, you might think, *I really blew it, so I might as well not bother testing, since I know my blood sugar is going to be high anyway. Now I feel so guilty since I blew it, I might as well not exercise today,*" Dr. Guzman says. Instead, a healthier thought would be, *Well, I ate that cake and now I feel bad; I guess I'd better do my walk to make up for it.*

■ Set small goals. When you're depressed, it can be hard to take positive actions. So when you set out to make a change for the better, make it small—that way you'll have a success to enjoy rather than a failure to face, Dr. Guzman says. "I might say, 'If you're currently doing nothing,

Joan, what do you think about walking around the block two or three times this week?' Then I help her visualize it: 'When would you do it? What would be your first step?' A lot of times people will set goals really big: 'I can walk every day,' and then they don't do it. When we start with a failure experience, it's not terribly motivating."

■ Forget the "shoulds." Turning a "should" such as "I should be able to follow a healthy meal plan every day" into an ironclad rule is unrealistic and doesn't leave room for mistakes, Dr. Guzman says. "A healthier belief would be, 'I'll do my best to follow a healthy meal plan, allowing for exceptions to the rule, and if I do make a mistake, I'll get right back on track.'"

■ Honor your successes. Make sure you celebrate your little successes and make them just as important to you as the things that don't go right, Dr. Guzman says. Feeling like the negative things count but the good ones don't is called disqualifying the positive. When you reach a goal, even a small one, congratulate yourself. Be sure to tell your support network so they can cheer you on, too.

■ **GET YOUR SHARE OF SHUT-EYE.** It's common for people with depression to have trouble either falling asleep or staying asleep, Dr. Dreelin says. However, without adequate rest, you're less likely to handle stress well. In fact, one of the first issues she tries to address with clients is sleep problems. Her tips:

■ Avoid caffeine or alcohol in the evenings. Both can interfere with sleep.

■ Avoid stimulation before bedtime: Don't fret over life's problems that are best left for the daytime, and remove the television from your bedroom.

■ Talk to your doctor about using a medication that will help you sleep.

■ **REMEMBER WHAT HIGH BLOOD SUGAR CAN DO.** "Walking around with blood sugar over 200 is like feeling on the verge of getting the flu," Dr. Koch says. That's definitely not going to help your depression. So do your best to keep your blood sugar under control—and remember that if you feel dark when your blood sugar is high, lowering it will soothe your spirit, which is an immediate reward.

■ **LEARN COPING SKILLS.** Dr. Dreelin spends much of her time helping clients learn ways to comfort themselves when they're stressed without using the tool that people commonly reach for: food. Make a list of 10 things you can do to relieve your stress that *don't* involve digging deeply into a container of ice cream. Maybe you can call a friend, soak in a warm bath, or make a cup of herbal tea. Include options that you can do easily and inexpensively. One good stress-relieving method is progressive muscle relaxation (PMR), which is described on page 215.

■ **SPEAK UP FOR YOURSELF.** Certain problems in your life will require some creativity and assertiveness to solve, Dr. Koch says. These include friends and family cajoling you about what you're eating or, conversely, keeping tempting foods in sight. Don't suffer in silence! If you've had enough of people's suggestions about how you should handle your diabetes, politely tell them that you appreciate their help, but you have a good system for knowing what you can and can't eat. If your family insists on having sugary foods in the house, work out a compromise regarding which foods are allowed and where they'll be stored—ideally, out of your sight. A counselor or therapist can help you learn how to become more assertive and creative in dealing with challenges.

■ **BREAK THE CYCLE OF ISOLATION.** When you're feeling depressed, it's common to isolate yourself and stop seeing people and doing things you normally enjoy. But cutting yourself off from others will just make you feel worse, Dr. Guzman says. Even if you have to force yourself, go out and do the fun activities you participated in before your diabetes diagnosis, she recommends. You don't have to dive back into your social schedule with the previous intensity. Just set very small goals: Maybe you'll call one old friend this week, go see one movie, meet someone for lunch, or read 50 pages in a book. But do a little something to get back into your former routine.

BETTER ATTITUDE EQUALS BETTER DIABETES CONTROL

In a 2004 study from the Medical College of Georgia, researchers interviewed 44 people with diabetes, then compared differences in attitudes between the 25 percent with the best blood sugar control and the 25 percent with the worst control. They described the people with the best control as committed or tentative.

■ Committed: After their diagnosis, these people didn't spend much time grieving about diabetes. They approached their diets with discipline and were generally committed to exercising. They measured their blood sugar regularly and considered their doctors to be partners in their efforts. Finally, they were determined to "do everything possible to live long and productive lives."

■ Tentative: These people were unhappier about having to deal with diabetes. They followed healthy eating habits, but while they were committed to managing the disease, they weren't yet doing all they could to control it.

The authors described the people with poorest control as hopeful, hassled, and overwhelmed.

■ Hopeful: These people were hopeful that if they could do self-care strategies, they could control their disease. However, most followed their previous eating habits and typically didn't exercise. They knew they needed to make major changes in order to manage their disease.

■ Hassled: These people were angry about their diagnosis. They practiced minimal self-care and felt that managing their diabetes would interfere with their lives.

■ Overwhelmed: These people put a low priority on their diabetes management and many had experienced complications. They didn't believe that self-care would help prevent problems, and they felt that they had little control over their health.

Do you see your attitudes among any of these groups? If your outlook on diabetes is more likely to contribute to poor blood sugar control, talk to your doctor, diabetes educator, or counselor about improving your "diatitude" to help keep yourself healthy despite your diabetes.

■ **SEEK PROFESSIONAL HELP.** "Some literature suggests that depression is harder to treat in people with diabetes than in nondiabetics," Dr. Dreelin says. "I've found that medication is very often necessary to produce significant change." Talk to your doctor about whether you would benefit from taking an antidepressant or antianxiety medication. If so, it's wise to combine the medication with sessions of cognitive-behavioral therapy—ideally, from a professional who understands diabetes, she says.

INDEX

Underscored page references indicate boxed text.

A

A1C test, 31, 64, 241–42, 248, 250, <u>251</u>
ABCs of diabetes, 42–43, 56–57, 175
Abdominal fat
  assessing, 159, 195
  body mass index and, 158
  body shapes and, 157
  health problems related to, 157–59
  insulin resistance and, 195
  liver disease and, 73
  medical terms for, 158
  metabolic syndrome and, 158, 160
  polycystic ovary syndrome and, 145
  preventing
    diet, 160–63
    exercise, 161, 180–81
    tips, 159–63
  smoking and, 159–60
  waist-to-hip ratio and, 158
ABI, <u>97</u>, 108
Accumin test, <u>67</u>
ACE inhibitors, <u>57</u>, 58, 67
Acetaminophen, 75
Acetyl-L-carnitine, 303
Adiponectin, 158
Aerobic exercise, 161, 179, 328
Age, 5–6, 17, 96, 236
Airline security and medications, <u>230</u>
Airplane food, avoiding, 229
Air pollution, avoiding, 172–74
Airport food, avoiding, 229–30
ALA, 304
Albumin levels, 64
Alcohol
  eating before imbibing, 169
  eating out and, 168–69
  gum disease and, 42
  liver disease and, 74–75
  stroke and, 153
Alpha-glucosidase inhibitors, 260
Alpha-lipoic acid (ALA), 304
Alprostadil, 92
Alzheimer's disease, 183

AmLactin, 110
Androgens, 141
Angioplasty, 104
Angiotensin-converting enzyme
    (ACE) inhibitors, <u>57</u>, 58, 67
Angiotensin II receptor blockers
    (ARBs), <u>57</u>, 58, 67, <u>152</u>
Ankle-brachial index (ABI), <u>97</u>, 108
Anthocyanins, 33
Antioxidants, 33
Antiseizure medications, 132
Apple body shape, 157
Apples, 204
ARBs, <u>57</u>, 58, 67, <u>152</u>
Arteries. *See* Peripheral arterial
    disease (PAD)
Artificial sweeteners, <u>224</u>, 225
Aspartame, <u>224</u>
Aspirin, 75, 153
Atenolol, <u>152</u>
Athlete's foot, 111
Atridox, <u>41</u>
Attitude, positive, 327–33, <u>332</u>, 333

B

Bariatric surgery, <u>273</u>
Bars, diabetic, <u>297</u>
Beans, 291–92
Beer. *See* Alcohol
Belly fat. *See* Abdominal fat
Benecol, 285
Ben-Gay, 132–33
Beta-blockers, <u>57</u>
Beverages, 197–98, 223. *See also* Alcohol;
    Water intake
Biguanides, 260
Biofeedback therapy, 34–35, 81–82
Bladder problems, 76–82, <u>79</u>, <u>81</u>
Blindness, 28, 253
Blood pressure. *See also* High blood pressure;
    Low blood pressure
  diabetes and, 32, 52–53
  exercise and, 182

monitoring, 42, 58, _97_, 250
stroke and, 150–52
Blood sugar levels. _See also_ Glucose
  adjustments, 246–47
  diet in preventing high, 65, 68
  during daytime, 246
  exercise and, 179–80, 247, _321_
  gum disease and, 36–37, 40
  health problems related to high, 242–43
  heart disease and, 49
  hypoglycemia and, 122
  kidney disease and, 65
  log of, 246
  mini meals and, 43
  monitoring, 56, 65, 72–73, _121_, 241–44, _245_,
    246, 248, 330–31
  overweight and, 193–94
  patterns, 246
  peripheral arterial disease and, 96, 100–101
  positive attitude and control of, _332_
  professional help and, 247–48
  as risk factor of diabetes, 237
  sleep and, 184–85
  type 2 diabetes and, 204
  urinary incontinence and, 79–80
  vision problems and, 32
Blood tests, _97_
Blueberries, 33, 296
Body mass index (BMI), 73, 158, 195, 237–38,
  269–70, 272
Body shapes, 157
Borderline diabetes, 183
Bran, 290
Breastfeeding, _22_
Broccoli, _211_
Brown sugar, 225
Buffets, avoiding, 167–68
Bunions, 111
B vitamin folate, 292
Byetta, 264
Bypass surgery, 104

C

CAD, _87_, 96
Caffeine, 188, 296, 298
Calcium, 304–5
Calluses, 111
Calorie needs, 195–96
Cancer, 146
Carbohydrates, 160–61, 166–67, 204,
  279–83, 287, 296
Cardiovascular exercise. _See_ Aerobic exercise
Cardiovascular system, 26–28.
    See also Heart disease
Carvedilol, _57_
Cataracts, _31_, _34_, 254
Celery, 205
CGMS, _121_, _245_

Cherries, 204
Chocolate, dark, 223
Cholesterol levels
  exercise and, 182–83
  HDL, _20_, 50, 294
  heart disease and, 50
  kidney disease and, 68
  LDL, _20_, 50, 260, 283, 285, 294
  liver disease and, 74
  metabolic syndrome and, _20_
  monitoring, 250–51
  peripheral arterial disease and, 96
  polycystic ovary syndrome and, 146
  stroke and, 151–52
Chromium, 305, 307
Cialis, 91
Cigarettes. _See_ Smoking
Cinnamon, 307–8
Circadian rhythm, _189_
Cirrhosis, 69–70, 75
Coenzyme Q10, 42
Coffee, 296, 298
Cognitive-behavioral therapy, 216–18, 329–30
Cold, avoiding, 172
Continuous glucose monitoring system
    (CGMS), _47_, _121_
Continuous positive airway pressure (CPAP), 187
Coping skills, learning, 331
Corn, 291
Corns, 111
Coronary artery disease (CAD), _87_, 96
Cortisol, 185
CPAP, 187
Cravings, managing, 221
Creatinine, 64
Cymbalta, 132

D

Dairy products, low-fat, 163, 292–93.
    See also specific type
Dark chocolate, 223
DASH diet, 57–58
Dehydration, 231
Dental care and exams, 41–42, _43_, _255_
Depression, 233, 239–40, 328–31
Desserts, 169, 221–22. _See also_ Sweets
DHA, 153–54, 310
DHEA (dehydroepiandrosterone), 93
Diabesity concept, 8–9
Diabetes. _See also specific complication and type_
  ABCs of, 42–43, 56–57, 175
  blood pressure and, 32, 52–53
  "community power" and, 13
  defining, 14–15
  diet in preventing, 239
  emotional issues associated with diagnosis of,
    3–5
  exercise in preventing, 178–83

Diabetes. *See also specific complication and type* (cont.)
expenditures spend on treating, 6
in future, 10–12
historical perspective of, 9
incidence and prevalence of, 5–7
information about, getting, 13, 327–28
as "lifestyle" disease, 8–9
manifestations, 23–24
reasons for rise in, 7–8
research, current, 24
risk factors
can be changed, 236–40
cannot be changed, 236
knowing, 101, 235
sleep and, 184–87
testing for, 19, 146
thrifty gene hypothesis and, 11
Diabetes food pyramid, 281
Diabetes meter, 232, 244
Diabetic bars and shakes, 297
Diabetic nephropathy, 125–34, 133, 135–37, 138–39
Diabetic retinopathy, 27–35, 31, 33, 34, 253–54
Diabetic ulcers, 106
Diet. *See also specific food*
balanced, 278–79
calorie needs and, 195–96
carbohydrates in, 160–61, 166–67, 204, 279–83, 287, 296
dairy products in, low-fat, 163, 292–93
DASH, 57–58
diabetes food pyramid and, 281
dietary fat in, 160, 275, 280, 284–85, 287, 288
eating out and, 164–69, 278
exercise and, 162
fiber in, 162, 197, 280, 283, 287, 291–92
food substitutions and, 295
glycemic index and, 49–50, 286, 292
grazing and, 203
Mediterranean, 73–74, 160
mini meals and, 43
plans, 51
plate method and, 287
in preventing
abdominal fat, 160–63
diabetes, 239
heart disease, 49–51
high blood pressure, 57–58
high blood sugar, 65, 68
hypoglycemia, 122–24
kidney disease, 68
liver disease, 73–74
overweight, 197–99
peripheral arterial disease, 102, 102
polycystic ovary syndrome, 145
stroke, 153–54
vision problems, 32–33
protein in, 68, 203–4, 280, 284
skipping meals, avoiding, 201–5

snacks, 204–5
sweets in, 219–23, 224, 225
trans fats in, avoiding, 275, 285
traveling and, 229–30
at work, 198
Dietary fat, 160, 275, 280, 284–85, 287, 288
Dieting, 197
Dining out, 164–69, 167, 278
Docosahexaenoic acid (DHA), 153–54, 310
D-Phenylalanine derivatives, 259
Dressings, salad, 168
Drugs. *See* Medications; *specific type*
Dry mouth, 41–42
Dry skin, 139

E

Eating out, 164–69, 167, 278
Eating times, 188, 202–3
ED, 83–93, 87, 89
Egg whites, 168
Eicosapentaenoic acid (EPA), 153–54, 310
Electromyography (EMG), 128
Emergencies, planning for, 232
EMG, 128
Endometrial cancer, 146
Endosperm, 290
Environmental exposure, 170–75
EPA, 153–54, 310
Epairestat, 133
Epigallocatechin gallate (EPCG), 313
Equal (artificial sugar), 224
Erectile dysfunction (ED), 83–93, 87, 89
Ethnicity as risk factor, 5, 7, 96, 154, 236
Exenatide, 264
Exercise. *See also* Walking
aerobic, 161, 179, 328
amount of, 178
blood pressure and, 182
blood sugar levels and, 179–80, 247, 321
cholesterol levels and, 182–83
classes, 200
diet and, 162
FITT model of, 98–99
fun and, 320–22
guidelines, 325–26
of hips, 199
importance of, 314
incremental, 199, 315–17, 316, 318
intensity of, 161
Kegel, 80–81
lack of, 8–9, 96, 176–83, 238
medical care before starting program of, 161
mental health and, 183
mood and, 183
muscle building and, 183–84
in preventing
abdominal fat, 161, 180–81
depression, 328–29

diabetes, 178–83
 heart disease, 51–52
 high blood pressure, 60, 182
 hypoglycemia, 322–25
 overweight, 199–200, 275
 peripheral arterial disease, 103
 polycystic ovary syndrome, 146
 stroke, 154
resistance training, 180, 200, 317, <u>318</u>
scheduling, 322
selecting appropriate, 319–20
of shoulders, 199
sleep and, 189–90
strength training, 180, 200, 317, <u>318</u>
tai chi, 189–90
traveling and, 228–31
type 2 diabetes and, 179–80
weight lifting, 180, 200, 317, <u>318</u>
for weight loss, 277
yoga, 189–90
Eye care and exams, 32, 253–55. *See also* Vision
 problems

F

Family medical history, 236
Fast food, avoiding, 231–32, <u>300</u>
Fasting glucose test, <u>19</u>
Fat. *See* Dietary fat; Abdominal fat; Obesity;
 Overweight
Fatty liver disease, 69–70, <u>72</u>
Fenofibrate, <u>33</u>
Fenugreek, 308–10
Fiber, 162, 197, 280, 283, 287, 291–92
Fish oils, 60, 310
FITT model of exercise, <u>98–99</u>
Focal photocoagulation, 35
Folate, 292
Food pyramid, diabetes, <u>281</u>
Foot care and exams, 59–60, 108, 110, <u>110</u>, 128,
 251–53
Foot problems, 105–13, <u>114</u>
Foot temperature, <u>110</u>
Foot ulcers, <u>110</u>
Fried foods, avoiding, 169
Frostbite, 172
Fruit, spreadable, 225
Fruits, 33, 160, 222. *See also specific type*
Fucoxanthin, 163
Fungal nails, 111

G

Gastrointestinal (GI) dysfunction, 138
Gender as risk factor, 5, 96, 237
Genetics, 18
Germ, 290
Gestational diabetes, 20–23, <u>22</u>
GFR, 64

GI dysfunction, 138
Ginseng, American, 92–93, 311
Glaucoma, <u>31</u>, 35, 254–55
Glomerular filtration rate (GFR), 64
Glucagon, 121–22
Glucose. *See also* Blood sugar levels
 breastfeeding and, <u>22</u>
 cortisol and, 185
 insulin and, 14–15
 monitoring, 65, <u>121</u>, 232, 241–44, 267
 tolerance test, <u>19</u>, 20
Glycemic index, 49–50, <u>286</u>, 292
Grazing, 203
Green tea, 298–99
Gum disease, 36–43, <u>40</u>, <u>41</u>, <u>43</u>
Gurmar, 225
Gymnema, 311–12
Gymnema sylvestre, 225

H

Hammertoes, 111–12
Hazardous environments, avoiding, 174
Health insurance, 244
Heart disease, 44–52, <u>47</u>, <u>49</u>, <u>51</u>, 152–53
Heat, avoiding, 172, 174–75
Hepatocyte growth factor (HGF), <u>34</u>
Herbal remedies, 92–93, 134, <u>135–37</u>.
 See also specific type
HGF, <u>34</u>
High blood pressure, 52–60, <u>55</u>, <u>57</u>, <u>59</u>, 66–67,
 96, 182
High cholesterol, peripheral arterial disease and,
 96
High heels, <u>114</u>
Hirsutism, 141
Homocysteine, 292
Hormone replacement therapy (HRT), 82, 92, 267
Hormone therapy, 82, 92
HRT, 82, 92, 267
HumaPen Memoir, 265
Hydration, 82, 168, 174, 188, 231
Hypertension, 52–60, <u>55</u>, <u>57</u>, <u>59</u>, 66–67, 96, 182
Hypoglycemia, 116–24
 breastfeeding and, <u>22</u>
 diabetic neuropathy and, 139
 exercise in preventing, 322–25
 insulin overdose and, <u>245</u>
 medical care for, <u>119</u>
 unawareness, <u>123</u>
Hypothermia, 172

I

Ibuprofen, 75
Immunizations, 251
Impotence, 83–93, <u>87</u>, <u>89</u>
Infections, bladder, 80
Inflammation, 10, <u>49</u>

Ingrown toenails, 112
Injections, 262–65
Injection therapy, 92
Insomnia, 184, 188
Insulin
    after childbirth, 22
    delivery devices, 265
    glucose and, 14–15
    impaired, 10, 15–16
    injections, 262–65
    pens, 265
    pumps, 265
    resistance, 21, 44–45, 70, 142, 179,
        195, 203
    traveling and dosages of, 232
Insulin-assisting agents, 260
Insulin-augmenting agents, 259
Insulin-sensitizing agents, 260–61
Insurance, health, 244
Intraurethral suppositories, 92
Iron, 173
Ischemia, 103–4
Isolation, avoiding, 331

J

Jelly, 225
Juvenile diabetes, 16. See also Type 1 diabetes

K

Kegel exercises, 80–81
Kelp, 163
Keralac, 110
Ketoacidosis, 243
Kidney disease, 61–68, 65, 67
Kidney function, 59, 251

L

Lactose intolerance, 293
Laser therapy, 35
Legumes, 291–92
Levitra, 91
Lidoderm, 133
Lifestyle changes, 236–40, 270.
        See also Diet; Exercise
Liposuction, 159
Liqiang 4, 309
Liver disease, 69–75, 72
Losartan, 152
Low blood pressure, 138

M

Macroplastique implants, 81
Macular edema, 31, 33
Magnesium, 60, 312–13
Margarine, 285

Medical care
    for erectile dysfunction, 89
    for exercise program, starting, 161
    for gum disease, 40
    for heart disease, 47
    for high blood pressure, 55
    for hypoglycemia, 119
    for kidney disease, 65
    for liver disease, 72
    medication list and, 253
    for peripheral arterial disease, 97
    for polycystic ovary syndrome, 143
    on regular basis, 249–56, 251, 266
    for stroke, 150
    for urinary incontinence, 79
    for vision problems, 31
MedicAlert bracelet, 123
Medical history, 96
Medications. See also specific type
    airline security and, 230
    carrying list of, 267
    in development, 262
    for diabetic neuropathy, 133
    eating out and, 167
    for erectile dysfunction, 91–93
    errors with, avoiding, 266–67
    extra dosages of, 261
    following directions and, 257–58, 267
    for high blood pressure, 57, 58
    injections, 262–65
    labels, reading, 267
    log of, 267
    by mail, 267–68
    medical care and list of, 253
    oral, 258–62
    pain relievers, OTC, 75
    for peripheral arterial disease, 103
    pharmacy and, 266–67
    reducing need for, 268
    skimping, 261
    skipping, 261
    storing, 268
    for stroke, 103, 151–52
    weight-loss, 276–77
Mediterranean diet, 73–74, 160
Meglitinides, 259
Melons, 205
Mental health and exercise, 183
Metabolically obese but normal weight (MONW),
        272
Metabolic syndrome, 20, 158, 160, 238–39
Metformin, 178, 195, 2602
Metoprolol, 57
Microalbuminuria test, 64
Microvascular complications, 66
Minerals, 135. See also specific type
Monofilament test, 108
Monounsaturated fats, 160
MONW, 272

Mood and exercise, 183
Muscle, building, 181
Music, listening to, 190

N

Nails, fungal, 111
Napping, 189
Neovascularization, 28
Nerve compression surgery, 133–34
Nerve conduction study, 128
Neuropathy, 106
Night-lights, avoiding, 190–91
Night shift, 185
Nonalcoholic fatty liver, 69, 72, 73
Nonnarcotic painkillers, 132
Nonproliferative retinopathy, 28
Nonsteroidal anti-inflammatory drugs (NSAIDs), 132
Nut butters, 294–95
NutraSweet, 224
Nutritionist, 50, 202–3
Nuts, 33, 205, 294–95

O

Oats, 291
Obesity, 8, 12, 17, 51, 96, 237–38
Olive oil, 288
Omega-3 fatty acids, 32–33, 153–54, 285
Omega-6 fatty acids, 33
Oral care and exams, 41–42, 43, 255
Oral medications, 260–64
Oranges, 204
OTCs, 75, 110, 132–33, 267
Overflow incontinence, 77, 80
Overweight
    assessing, 195
    blood sugar levels and, 193–94
    incidence of, 192–93
    lifestyle and, 12
    perceptions of, 192–93
    preventing
        diet, 197–99
        exercise, 199–200, 275
        walking, 200
    type 2 diabetes and, 17–18

P

PAD, 94–96, 98–99, 101, 102, 106–7, 149
Pain relievers, OTC, 77
Panretinal photocoagulation, 35
PCOS, 140–46, 143
PDE inhibitors, 91
Pear body shape, 157
PEDF, 34
Pedometer, 321
Penile prosthesis, 92
Performance anxiety, alleviating, 90

Periodontitis, 36–43, 40, 41, 43
Periostat, 41
Peripheral arterial disease (PAD), 94–96, 98–99, 101, 102, 106–7, 149
Peripheral vision check, 255
Phosphodiesterase (PDE) inhibitors, 91
Photocoagulation, 35
Physical exams, 97. See also Medical care
Pigment epithelium derived factor (PEDF), 34
Plantar warts, 112
Plate method, 287
Podiatrist, 252
Polycystic ovary syndrome (PCOS), 140–46, 143
Popcorn, air-popped, 205
Portions, 198, 287–88, 294
Positive attitude, 327–33, 332, 333
Posture, nighttime, 191
Pramlintide, 264
Prediabetes, 6, 18–20, 19, 179
Pregnancy, 20–23
Prescriptions. See Medications; specific type
Processed and packaged food, avoiding, 300
Professional help, seeking, 50, 191, 247–48, 333. See also Cognitive-behavioral therapy; Medical care
Progressive muscle relaxation, 215–16
Proliferative retinopathy, 30–31, 31, 33
Promise Activ, 285
Propionyl-L-carnitine, 92–93
Protein, 68, 203–4, 280, 284, 287
Protein bars, 205
Protein kinase C beta enzyme, 62
Pulse checks, 97

Q

Quantitative sensory testing (QST), 128

R

Race as risk factor, 5, 7, 96, 154, 236
Refined grains, 290
Relaxation, 34–35
Resistance training, 180, 200, 317, 318
Restless leg syndrome, 184
Retinal detachment, 28, 31, 31
Revascularization, 104
Risk factors of diabetes. See also specific factor
    can be changed, 236–40
    cannot be changed, 236
    knowing, 101, 235
Roughage, 162, 197, 280, 283, 287
Rule of 15s, 120–21
Rye, 291

S

Saccharin, 224
Salt, 58–59, 153

Saturated fats, 285
Scale, weight, 196
Scatter photocoagulation, 35
Screenings, regular, 249–56, <u>253</u>. *See also specific type of test*
Seaweed, 163
Secondhand smoke, 175, <u>209</u>
Sedentary lifestyle, 8–9, 96, 176–83, 238
Selenium, <u>306</u>
Self-care, 266, 329
Serving sizes, 198, 294
Sex dysfunction, <u>9</u>, 83–93, <u>87</u>
Shakes, diabetic, <u>297</u>
Shoes, 113, <u>114</u>, 115, <u>324</u>
Sildenafil, 91
Skin softeners, 110
Skipping meals, avoiding, 201–5
Sleep
    amount of, trend, 184
    assessing personal amount of, 187–88
    blood sugar levels and, 184–85
    circadian rhythm and, <u>189</u>
    cortisol and, 185
    counseling for improving, 191
    depression and, 330
    diabetes and, 184–87
    exercise and, 189–90
    lack of, 184–91
    napping and, <u>189</u>
    need for, 184–85
    night shift and, <u>185</u>
    optimum, 185
    posture at night and, 191
    problems, 184
    restless leg syndrome and, 184
    smoking and, 190
    tips for improving, 188–91
    traveling and, 227–28
    walking and, 190
Sleep apnea, 184
Smoking
    abdominal fat and, 159–60
    broccoli and, <u>211</u>
    gum disease and, 42
    health problems related to, 206–12, 239
    heart disease and, 51
    kidney disease and, 68
    peripheral arterial disease and, 96
    as risk factor of diabetes, 239
    secondhand, 175, <u>209</u>
    sleep and, 190
    stroke and, 153
    tips for quitting, 208–12
    weight loss and, 275–76
Snacks, 204–5, 229
Social determinants, 12
Soda, 197–98, 223
Sodium, 58–59, 153

Soy yogurt, 295–96
Splenda, <u>224</u>
Stevia, 225
Strength training, 180, 200, 317, <u>318</u>
Stress, 173–74, 185, 213–18
Stress incontinence, 77, <u>81</u>
Stroke, 147–54, <u>150</u>, <u>152</u>, <u>154</u>
Sucralose, <u>224</u>
Sugar alcohols, <u>224</u>
Sugars, 145, 225
Sugar Twin, <u>224</u>
Sulfonylureas, 259
Supplements, 60, 304–5. *See also specific type*
Support, social, 13, 89, 123, 210, 328
Surgical treatments. *See specific type*
Sweet'N Low, <u>224</u>
Sweets, 219–23, <u>224</u>, 225. *See also* Desserts
Symlin, 264

T

Tadalafil, 91
Tai chi, 189–90
Tea, green, 298–99
TENS, 133
Testosterone replacement, 92
Thiazolidinediones, 260–61
Thrifty gene hypothesis, <u>11</u>
Toothpaste, 42
Topical creams and patches, 132–33
Transcutaneous electrical nerve stimulation (TENS), 133
Trans fats, 275, 285
Traveling, 226–32, <u>230</u>
Tricyclic antidepressants, 132
Triglyceride levels, 260
Tylenol, 75
Type 1 diabetes. *See also specific complication*
    age risk factor and, 236
    breastfeeding and, <u>22</u>
    causes of, 170–71
    defining, 15–16
    ethnicity and, 236
    insulin pumps and, 265
    kidney disease and, 63
    symptoms, 15
Type 2 diabetes. *See also specific complication*
    age risk factor and, 17, 236
    blood sugar levels and, 204
    breastfeeding and, <u>22</u>
    defining, 16–18
    ethnicity and, 236
    exercise and, 179–80
    insulin pumps and, 265
    insulin resistance and, 44–45, 179
    kidney disease and, 63
    as "lifestyle" disease, 8–9
    liver disease and, 69–70

obesity and, 8, 17
overweight and, 17–18
symptoms, 17

U

Ulcers, 106, <u>110</u>
Ultrasound, 128
Unsaturated fats, 285
Urge incontinence, 77, 81
Urinary incontinence, 76–82, <u>79</u>, <u>81</u>, 138

V

Vaccinations, 251
Vacuum constriction devices, 92
Vardenafil, 91
Vascular endothelial growth factor (VEGF), 28, <u>34</u>
Vegetables, 169. *See also specific type*
VEGF, 28, <u>34</u>
Viagra, 91
Vibration perception threshold (VPT), 108
Vinegar, 299, 301
Vision problems, 27–35, <u>31</u>, <u>33</u>, <u>34</u>, 138–39, 253–55
Visual acuity test, 254
Vitamin C, 42
Vitamin D, 304–5
Vitamins, <u>137</u>. *See also specific type*
Vitrectomy, 35
Volatile organic compounds (VOCs), 175
VPT, 108

W

Waist circumference, 271–72, 275
Waist-to-hip ratio (WHR), 158
Wakame, 163
Walking
  after meal, 200
  pedometer and, 321
  in preventing
    overweight, 200
    peripheral arterial disease, 103

shoes, <u>324</u>
sleep and, 190
traveling and, 228–29, 231
Warts, plantar, 112
Water intake, 82, 168, 174, 188, 231
Water pollution, avoiding, 174
Weighing self, 196
Weight lifting, 180, 200, 317, <u>318</u>
Weight loss. *See also* Abdominal fat, tips for reducing
  body mass index and, 269–70, 272
  exercise for, 277
  facts about, 269–70
  goals, 196
  health benefits of, 194–95
  medications for, <u>276–77</u>
  metabolically obese but normal weight and, 272
  motivation for, 196
  in preventing
    heart disease, <u>51</u>
    kidney disease, 67–68
    liver disease, 73
    polycystic ovary syndrome, 144–45
    urinary incontinence, 80
  smoking and, 275–76
  surgery for, <u>273</u>
  tips for, 275–77
  waist circumference and, 271–72, 277
Weight maintenance, healthy, 73, 80
Wheat, 291
Whole grains, 205, 289–91
WHR, 158
Wine. *See* Alcohol
Work, <u>185</u>, 198
Wound care, 112–13

Y

Yoga, 189–90
Yogurt, 293, 295–96
Yohimbe, 93